Praise for

"By turns witty, vivid, and harrowing, *Rewriting Illness* reads as though Nora Ephron had written a book called *I Feel Bad About My Tumor*. Especially good on the abrupt, stopped-time feeling when the flow of life—city life, complicated life, sentient life—collides with illness." —THOMAS BELLER, author of *J .D. Salinger: The Escape Artist* (winner, New York City Book Award for Biography/Memoir)

"It's not courage unless you're afraid, and Elizabeth Benedict has courage—and fear—in abundance, in this frank, riveting and often hilarious memoir. If you've had cancer, or love someone who's had or has it, or are just plain afraid of it—that's to say pretty much everyone— then you'll want to read this book." —CLAIRE MESSUD, author of *The Emperor's Children, The Woman Upstairs*, and *The Burning Girl*

"Memoirs of serious illness are often good suspense stories, and this one is a page-turner. I read Elizabeth Benedict's *Rewriting Illness* in a single sitting and finished it infinitely more knowledgeable about what it means to be diagnosed with cancer. Here is someone who's figured out not only how to think about the unthinkable but how to turn her experience into an honest, gripping, and genuinely humorous story. It's the kind of inspiring book you want to share with all the important people in your life." —SIGRID NUNEZ, author of *What Are You Going Through* and *The Friend: A Novel* (2018 National Book Award for Fiction)

"I thought I wasn't a fearful person, and then I read *Rewriting Illness*. Sleeping alone in the country (not the city—lots of people around to hear me scream). Picking up my car late at night in a parking lot. My fears aren't particularly rational—how many ax murderers are there, and what are the chances one will cross my path? Elizabeth's Benedict's beautiful, brave memoir about her own fears, especially fear of illness, which was eventually realized and had to be overcome, has so much to say about rational and irrational anxieties and the way they haunt women and deprive us of the larger life we crave." —KATHA POLLITT, author of *Learning to Drive: And Other Life Stories* and *Subject to Debate: Sense and Dissents on Women, Politics and Culture*

"*Rewriting Illness* is a superbly intelligent and surprisingly entertaining memoir about what happens when a lifelong fear of illness collides at last with illness itself. Elizabeth Benedict applies her formidable talents as a novelist to bringing to life the scenes and characters from her *annus horribilis* dealing with lymphoma. She writes with an honesty and a sly sense of humor about herself that make this book hard to put down." —STEPHEN MCCAULEY, author of *My Ex-Life*

"The moment every woman dreads of finding a lump where no lump should be is the jumping off point for Elizabeth Benedict's startling, self-aware, and wickedly funny memoir. Whether she's describing her sister teaching her Tibetan chants to calm her nerves, the big city doctors who dismiss her concerns, or her problems with Susan Sontag's cancer metaphor critique, Benedict brings a novelist's deft storytelling to a narrative we think we already know. It's full of drama, humor, essential lessons for dealing with doctors, crushing vulnerability and— wonderfully—plenty of hope." —MARA LIASSON, NPR, national political correspondent

"I devoured Elizabeth Benedict's beautiful book in one sitting—truly couldn't put it down. I'm moved and astonished by how she made her cancer story universal, even for someone who is not yet, knock wood, a member of that club. Brava for this forthright and fascinating account." —BETSY WEST, documentary director, *RBG, Julia,* and *Gabby Giffords Won't Back Down*

"Nuanced, thoughtful, with not a cliché in sigh. Impossible to put down because the rich inner life of the writer—this excellent writer— is so compelling. The story she tells—vividly, in fits and starts, as it happened—is a reflection of encountering the unpredictable vicissitudes of life, and its one certainty." —KATHERINE DALSIMER, Weill Cornell Medical College; author of *Virginia Woolf: Becoming a Writer* and *Female Adolescence: Psychoanalytic Reflections on Literature*

Rewriting
ILLNESS

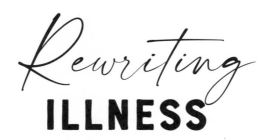

Rewriting ILLNESS

A VIEW OF MY OWN

ELIZABETH BENEDICT

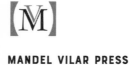

MANDEL VILAR PRESS

DRYAD PRESS

This book is typeset in Minion Pro. The paper used in this book meets the minimum requirements of ANSI/NISO Z39.48-1992 (R1997). ∞

Text designed by Barbara Werden

PUBLISHER'S CATALOGING-IN-PUBLICATION DATA
Name: Benedict, Elizabeth
Title: Rewriting Illness: A View of My Own
Description: Simsbury, Connecticut, Mandel Vilar Press [2023]
    Takoma, Maryland, Dryad Press [2023]
Identifiers: ISBN 978-1942134-916 (pbk.)
    E-ISBN 978-1942134-909 (ebook)
Subjects: Benedict, Elizabeth-Memoir, Cancer, Health—Hypochondria—Tumor—
    Cancer Diagnosis—Lymphoma—United States—Autobiography—Diagnosis—
    Treatments—Dealing with Doctors—New York City—21st Century Women
    Writers—American—Medical—Personal Memoirs
Classification LCC RC280 B9 2023

Printed in the United States of America
23 22 23 24 25 26 27 28 29 / 9 8 7 6 5 4 3 2 1

MANDEL VILAR PRESS
Simsbury, Connecticut
and
DRYAD PRESS
Takoma Park, Maryland

www.americasforconservation.org | www.mvpublishers.org

For James and Emily

"I learned about a lot of things in medical school, but
mortality wasn't one of them."
DR. ATUL GAWANDE, *Being Mortal*

"I am always on the phone, always writing letters, always waking
up to address myself to B. and D. and C.—those whom
I dare not ring up until morning and yet must talk
to throughout the night."
ELIZABETH HARDWICK, *Sleepless Nights*

Rewriting
ILLNESS

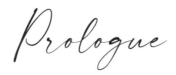

Wish You Were Here

Fear is inventive.

Cancer is not contagious.

Brain cells can regenerate.

Silence is not merely the absence of sound.

Anxiety is not equally apportioned between the sexes.

Adaptation is a biological process by which organisms or species become better suited to their environments.

Years after her diagnosis in 1975 of stage four breast cancer, Susan Sontag wrote, "I am gleaming with survivorship."

According to many studies on happiness, including the most popular course ever taught at Yale, and later taken online by three million people, individuals who exercise daily, do things for others, and take regular note of what they have to be grateful for are happier than those who don't. And, I would add, people who are in close touch with others. Which must mean that with all the ways we have to be in touch in the twenty-first century, happiness is on the rise and loneliness on the decline.

Do kids who've grown up with computers, smart phones, and texting know what it means to be out of touch for days, sometimes weeks? Do they know a "long-distance phone call" used to be so expensive these calls were often special occasions? Do they know that people on vacation sent postcards—many, many postcards—to friends and loved ones because there was no other way to be in touch? Can they picture travelers sitting in cafés with a half dozen postcards, writing out messages and then having to figure how and where to get stamps, which was sometimes so difficult they came home with a batch of unsent cards, tiny messages, little kisses, *See you soon's* and *Wish you were here's*.

I can't think about all those postcards and letters without remembering how much loneliness there was in those days, so much distance between us, and no other way to measure it except in time: the time it takes for a postcard or a letter to travel from point A to point B, the time that will elapse before X will see Y again. And measured in the phrase—with words of one syllable, words of so few letters: *I miss you so much*.

My husband sometimes texts me from the bedroom, two rooms from where I am in the living room. On the other side of the apartment, he reads, listens to music, and prepares his classes. *Nap*, he sometimes texts or, *Doing laundry tonight*.

Sometimes I text him: *Do you want a visitor?*

When cell phones were firmly a feature of most lives, my sister said that it would have been wonderful to have had one in the late 1970s and early '80s when she was living with an Italian man who often didn't talk much, except to his friends late at night in their tiny apartment, when she was trying to sleep. *I could have walked down the street with him and called Suki, and it would have made such a difference. I would have been much less lonely.*

When I found true love with the man who texts me from the bedroom, I replaced years of loneliness with fears that I added to the small collection of large fears I already had. Now at the top of the list is the fear that I will lose the true love because he will die or I will die. When my cell phone rings and I don't recognize the number, I'm afraid it's a stranger calling to tell me that my husband is in the hospital. He had an accident or a heart attack, and I have to get there right away. Or I'm already too late. Every night as I brush my teeth, I think: *We made it through another day without dying.*

It feels like an achievement because in an ordinary day of several phone calls from unfamiliar numbers, I come so close to losing him.

I would miss you so much.

PART
One

Cookies and Milk

Might it have been Sue Briskman who made me a hypochondriac? The way she sat on the battered couch in our senior lounge, where we twenty-two Lenox girls congregated between classes, and complained about a lump on the underside of her chin? The way, a month later, she said she had to have blue dye shot into her feet so the doctors could see what was going on in her body. And the way not long after—February 24, 1972, to be exact—she had the audacity to depart this world at seventeen years old, felled by something called Hodgkin's disease, which one of the girls explained to me as news spread through the school: "You get bumps all over your body. It's hideous. And then you die."

An hour earlier, I had been alone in the school library on the fourth floor, where I often luxuriated in free periods, reading about the Lost Generation. When I noticed it was eleven o'clock, I trotted down to the cafeteria in the basement for our morning infusion of cookies and milk. Nothing seemed out of place until an eleventh grader sitting across from me said, "Are you upset?"

A curious question. I was often annoyed by one thing or another when not swaddled in a cloud of melancholy, but how would she know that? "About what?"

"Sue died this morning. Didn't you hear?"

I managed to shake my head as it nearly short-circuited with shock. Wasn't she just getting some tests . . . Hadn't she just . . . My lips went numb.

I staggered upstairs and heard that classes were canceled, and when I passed a friend of Sue's in the narrow back stairwell, I asked, "Who's going to the funeral?" She spun around and glared at me.

"Everyone. Aren't you?" I hadn't planned to, but the intensity of the glare made me reconsider. I barely knew Sue and had little to say to her clique of friends, the long-haired girls who'd been together since first grade, lived in lavish apartments, and had never been on the subway or below 59th Street. But the next morning, I took the bus across Central Park and squeezed into the end of a row in the mobbed chapel at Riverside Memorial, moments before the service began. Our class filled two rows to the sounds of whispers, sniffles, and charm bracelets tinkling against silk-lined winter coats coming off. I had never spoken a word to Sue, but I could not bear more than a glance at the casket, her grand wooden box engulfed in grief, parked at the altar. How many funerals had any of us been to at that point? It was only my second.

Tears began to flow a few sentences into the rabbi's sermon as a stack of tissues came down the row. I was determined not to cry, but I took one and squeezed it until it absorbed the sweat of my palm. A massive lump rose in my throat as the rabbi quoted the Bible and talked about Sue's youth. I could hear the girl next to me struggle to hold back sobs, but I did not know to put my arm around her or touch her clenched hand, any of the gestures I would make now, even to a stranger, much less a girl who had been in school with Sue since first grade.

Walking by the elegant stone school building as I do now about once a year, I'm flooded with memories and waves of gratitude. After an early lifetime in the rough and tumble of New York City public schools, I spent my last two years of high school there, in classes of eight or twelve or twenty girls, taught by women with the luxury to engage in subjects they had studied at Vassar and Bryn Mawr. The contrast was stark: in our apartment fifteen blocks uptown, my parents' rocky marriage was unraveling in a brutal fashion, but in the school's nineteenth-century townhouse, I was pampered with attention, lavished with books, made to believe that I should take myself seriously. But I still cannot walk down that street without thinking of how Sue's death rewired my central nervous system, made me leap with fear at every bodily symptom and a good proportion of my medical encounters. From then on, my brain told me that I had to be vigilant, always on guard against the slightest anomaly.

My most vivid memories of Sue are in the senior lounge, where the entire class crammed happily into a space about six feet wide and ten feet long and waited for a slot on the old couch. We'd plop down talking and laughing in our matching navy herringbone skirts, cheek to cheek, like subway riders. I see Sue clearly, her petite frame, her long, thick dark brown hair parted down the middle in the Joan Baez style of the day, though Sue was no bohemian. In my memory, she wore a bit of gold jewelry, didn't say much in classes, and moved not with a swagger but an air of belonging. Heavy eyebrows and generally wispy looks went with her soft voice, as though she just might blow away. In not one memory is she talking to me, looking at me, though I was always, it seems, looking at her, or maybe I started staring once she'd made the announcement about the lump. I saw her only a few times after that. Above our matching skirts, we were allowed to wear any white blouse or top we pleased, and I see Sue in a ribbed white turtleneck, smiling, delicate, doomed. *There's a bump right here. I'm going to the doctor this afternoon.*

I would learn later that, because I had been in the library, I had missed being gathered into Mrs. K.'s office for the announcement.

Missed the details, the information about the funeral, the shared moment of astonishment and connection with the other girls, now that there were twenty-one of us.

Now It's Your Turn

That day I was out of the Sue loop, but in all the years since then, she has never been far outside mine. Decades passed, and when a Facebook page for our class appeared one day, I signed on. In 2012, I realized we were coming up on forty years since graduation, and through the page, I suggested a gathering. I wanted to know what had become of the twenty other women—and I had a lingering question for them.

Ten of us gathered at the East Side apartment of a classmate, and a few hours into the party, once we had shared stories of careers, families, and disappointments, I ventured a question: "I'm wondering if anyone has been haunted by Sue's death?" As I looked around the table, I was silently stunned by the heads shaking calmly. Barely a flutter. No one mentioned a single lingering effect. The woman who had been Sue's closest friend was not there, but on that night of backward glances, my conversational gambit went nowhere. I had barely known the girl, and yet she had lurked in my consciousness, always prepared to pounce and shout, "Boo!" And, "Now it's your turn!"

Five years after the reunion, late one night in early June 2017, after saying goodnight to a dear young friend who had come for dinner, I crossed my left arm over my chest and stuck it in my armpit, and there it was.

Man at the Door

For several weeks before, I had been feeling something weird inside what's called the shoulder girdle, a busy intersection, the convergence of several of the body's major highways. It was a vague sensation in the vicinity of the hinge of my underarm. Sometimes I was aware of it and mostly I wasn't, and when I noticed it, it never hurt. I hadn't thought to mention it to James or to touch it because I didn't think there would be anything to feel, it was so indistinct, as though it might have been a tiny pellet floating inside me.

The sensation of encountering a shape so definitive, so solid—when I had expected nothing—was an electric charge, a cartoon of a character putting her finger in a light socket. I knew in an instant that it could be gravely dangerous, like the proverbial man showing up at the door with a gun—Raymond Chandler's advice for how to create tension in a detective story. The gun was aimed right at me.

If I added up the hours I had spent anticipating the moment I'd feel a lump where no lump should be, it's the high two figures. I had never compared notes with friends about their levels of anxiety around this particular imaginary moment, but I knew my own fears were extreme. I braced, with the manic energy of a crazed Roz Chast character, for monthly self-breast exams, the daily exams leading up to the yearly mammograms, the nausea of waiting, back when we had to, for letters in the mail with their results, the pelvic exams, sonograms for this and that, and attempts to interpret the looks on the faces of technicians and doctors as they snapped pictures and pushed and pinched my insides. Weeks of worry, Mobius strips of fear.

I'm here to say that the moment turns out to be every bit as terrifying as I had always imagined it would be.

Not Everything Scares the Shit Out of Me

I do not want to leave the impression that cowering in fear is my reaction to all of life, when there is so much that rattles people that I am not afraid of. I am not afraid of blank pages, public speaking, public transportation, dinner parties, countries where I don't speak the language, interpersonal conflict, difficult conversations, sex, writing about sex, talking about sex in public, and explaining, in public, how to write a sex scene in a work of fiction. I mention sex in so many guises because of a book I was asked to write in 1994—writerly advice on what makes a good sex scene in a work of fiction—which came out two years later and has been in print ever since. I have been talking fearlessly about the subject for decades on stately radio stations, at literary conferences, and in writing workshops. People interviewing me are sometimes nervous or—I'm not sure—put on a show of it as they speak for many in the audience. The questions I often hear are: "But what if my mother reads what I write?" or "What should I call the body parts?" Not a single question has ever ruffled one of my feathers. But if my hand goes casually to my neck, and I sense anything remotely bumpy or out of place, I feel the threat in my knees in a nanosecond.

To go *weak in the knees*. To be taken over or pulled under by fear, this primal, primary emotion. When paired with a color, it would have to be red. A stop light, a stop sign, the color of emergency lights on a car. Fear is elemental, often irrational, and entirely necessary. Without a hearty dose of it, we're dead. With too much, we're paralyzed, agoraphobic. My mellow husband genuinely panics at the prospect of being late, even when visiting friends. When Susan Sontag learned she had cancer in 1975, she slept with the lights on, but years later, she went eleven times to Sarajevo in the midst of a war and directed a production of *Waiting for Godot*.

Drop a pin in the place on the map marked "Fear."

One Night I Touched My Arm

Seconds after I discovered the lump, I said aloud to myself, "What do I do now?" meaning that minute and for the rest of the night. It was eleven o'clock. James was in the bedroom, two rooms away, but I didn't call out to him immediately, didn't go into the bedroom and tell him because I wanted more information. He is the King of Calm, and I knew he would not entertain that this could be a crisis until he had it in writing. He would say, in the soothing tone of a pilot encountering turbulence, "Don't worry. You'll call the doctor first thing in the morning." And he would refuse to believe that I could be gravely ill— because look at me! Lucid, energetic, my usual self.

I listed to the laptop on the couch, which doubles as my desk, and Googled "reasons lump armpit." Cysts, temporarily swollen lymph nodes, lymphoma, or a warning sign that breast cancer was on its way, even if it had not yet arrived in the breast. The news was either pretty good, not great, or Get Your Affairs in Order.

This lump was brazen. It was asking for attention, and it had mine. All of it. I could not stop examining it, though my experience was nil and my tools, my fingers, primitive. But if I touched it enough, from every possible angle, couldn't it reveal its true nature to me? It was, after all, *right there*. It was round or roundish, and when I raised my arm above my head, it retreated, a ball into a billiard pocket. With my arm extended at shoulder height, I could push it around under the skin. It was not fixed to my ribcage. That had to be good, didn't it? Less fatal than a lump that stuck to another body part? Was this a question for Google? But even if Google knew, did I really want the answer?

Would I follow Sontag and sleep with the lights on?

Evanescent

The word, a favorite, crept into my head that night in the living room, right beside all the words about things that were not about to disappear. *Evanescent*. The joyful me who had buzzed around the living room five minutes before was gone. The moments of exquisite contentment and possibility were over: the euphoria of our dinner, the relief I'd felt for the last week, that there was no more drama in my life for a while: a week before, I had finished a difficult draft of a novel that had taken many years—and before those years, many decades of trying to figure out how I would disguise the story at the heart of it. The book was not done, but this draft had taken me to another level of certainty about what I was doing, and I had the summer and fall to write the next draft. I was three-quarters of the way up the mountain. I could almost see the summit.

Gone too in that searing moment was the joy I often felt when James was twenty feet away, in the bedroom, reading and probably listening to music on headphones, because music is the background to everything he does, except when it's the foreground, which is often—when he's listening to recordings, talking to or listening to his violinist daughter, Emily, or teaching people how to listen to music.

We had been together for almost twenty years, second marriages for each of us, and though I am not the mother of his Emily, I have been her dad's big love, and he has been mine, since she was twelve, and she knows that she is my other big love. She knows that in my first marriage, I had wanted to adopt a child from Vietnam, though she doesn't know the whole story.

She and her father connect around many subjects, but most intensively and intricately around music. When they talk about it, when they listen to it, when she plays, they escape into a world in which the rest of time stands still, and they exist only in the music. I had never known people who could shut off so much of the quotidian as James and Emily. I had never been close to people who could dwell so completely *in the moment*, even when the moment was an hour. I had spent a lifetime with writers, New Yorkers, kvetchers, people obsessed with the burdens of the past and the potential calamities of the future. We could stop for art, stop for sex, food, movies, and a dozen other activities, but there was always a sense that we were in a holding pattern before we could get back to what really mattered: worrying about what happened long ago and what might happen tomorrow. And complaining. But this was not the case when James and Emily huddled together on their island of music, swapping notes on octaves, cadenzas, and Arvo Pärt. Over the years, they've taught me about that kind of stillness and concentration, and I've taught them what I know—a cruder talent, or no talent at all: the exquisite joy of complaining.

Now I would have to interrupt James' songs, his reverie, his life and my own, with *this intruder*, this inelegant lump. The wonderful soundtrack of our lives—Bach, Beethoven, the Schumanns, the Elvises, Miles Davis, Bob Dylan, Aretha, gigabytes of classical, jazz, pop, and a little hip-hop—was about to go silent.

"Sweetie?" The first word I spoke once I heard James' footsteps in the next room, closer than he had been before. I was saddled now with this new identity. My run of good fortune had come to an end. In a handful of seconds, the plot had zigzagged in another direction, clear off the page. "Would you come in here? I have something to tell you."

A Handful of Seconds

He is tender, steady, and reasonable. "You'll call the doctor in the morning," he says. He keeps his shit together in exactly the way I expect he will. I know that if the situation were reversed, and he had just found a lump in his own body, our emotions would be identical: I would panic at the thought of losing him, and he would assure me that he is not going to die anytime soon.

He does not *do* panic. He tries to calm things down when emotions run high, and when faced with grief—his sister's diagnosis of stage four lung cancer, her death six years later—he holds things in rather than lets them out. He grew up in Amherst, Massachusetts, and he may have learned a thing or two about grieving from his ghostly neighbor, Emily Dickinson: "After great pain / a formal feeling comes"—as opposed, say, to having a baroque meltdown. It was a response conditioned too by his father, who had a terrible temper. James was the only one of five children and a mother who could say, "Dad, this is not helping the situation," and his father would sometimes snap out of it. But there were plenty of times when his father did not snap out of it, and James learned to endure the explosions and do what boys are taught to do: suck it up. Like a lot of men, he's reserved in his emotional expression, but, unlike a lot of men, he is tender and kind and talks often about the ways music and art work on our emotions, allow us to *feel* and discover our emotions. When we met in 1999— pioneers on an Internet dating site—we were the only people whose favorite movie was *My Night at Maud's*. I lived on the Upper West Side of Manhattan and he lived in the People's Republic of Cambridge. It was love at second email.

It took me a long time to get used to James' reserve after my first husband's emotional instability, the sadness that underlay even his high spirits and greatest joys: the death of his eighteen-year-old son a year before we met, probably a suicide. He was not afraid to cry. Disinclined to hide his emotions or freeze up, he could get weepy at TV commercials—the schmaltzy ones they play at the Super Bowl. In our relationship, I was the less emotional one, and we sometimes joked that we had our sex roles reversed.

James and I do a better job of performing our respective genders.

"Show me where it is," he said.

"It's hard to find." I held out my arm and tried to guide his fingers to the place, but the lump had a way of disappearing, and he was not used to poking around in anyone's armpit.

"That?" he said. "Is that it?"

"I think so."

"Does it hurt?"

"Not at all."

"I can't really tell much about it. But you'll find out tomorrow."

Yes, tomorrow and tomorrow and tomorrow.

Insurance

At 9:01 the next morning, I lunged for my phone and booked a noon appointment with Sylvie, the nurse practitioner who had essentially been my doctor for the last eight years. Sylvie the NP. Not her real name. My health insurance would pay for this visit, but just in case this lump was *It*, my next call was to my accountant, an essential player in the drama of saving my one and only wild and precious life.

As a hypochondriac—did I mention that I'm a hypochondriac?—and a lifelong freelancer used to buying my own health insurance, I am often forced to buy a different policy every year because of changing rules. And I had a manila file for just this possibility. I had made a deal with myself when I last signed up for insurance, the previous December: if I needed to—a euphemism for *got cancer*—I would incorporate my business and become eligible to buy much more expensive health insurance that covered out-of-network doctors. My accountant could file incorporation papers in four days, and once I filled out the forms and shelled out a vast sum of money, the new insurance would be effective the first of the following month—in this case, July first. If I hadn't had the money in the bank to pay the extra thousand dollars a month for the next six months, James and I would have raided our retirement accounts. If the lump was nothing serious, which I'd know in a New York minute, I could nix the new policy.

The pricey insurance, enabling me to go to any doctor and any hospital, was one of my get-out-of-jail-free cards. Another card was a longtime friendship with the former head of Memorial Sloan Kettering. I had always taken some comfort knowing I could contact him for guidance and referrals. But it was much too soon—I'd need more than a hypochondriac's hunch to play that card.

What the NP Said

"Wow! That's big!" said Sylvie. "You should get that looked at." A pause to collect herself after the shock of it. "It's probably a lymph node that's fighting off an infection. They sometimes take a month to go away."

She gave me a referral for a sonogram, and that Friday afternoon, I made an appointment for Monday at the East Side radiology clinic, a free-standing fear factory where I'd been getting mammograms for four years. They read the X-rays in ten minutes and tell you the results before you take off the hospital gown. And they take a raft of health insurances instead of just a chosen few, so I could keep going there.

I took comfort in Sylvie's diagnosis that I had a swollen lymph node, but my Monday appointment gave me the weekend to begin a campaign to shrink the thing. I studied natural remedies on the Internet and went with the simplest first: turmeric tea and Bragg Apple Cider Vinegar, downing as much as I could of both. And I confided in my sister, Nancy, and three close friends, including Deena Kolbert, an artist, entrepreneur, activist, WBAI radio show host, and life coach, who was also a thirty-eight-year breast cancer survivor. By the time doctors finally diagnosed her cancer, it had spread so far that she had to have twenty-eight lymph nodes removed.

Deena had survived two years of 1980s-vintage chemo and radiation by pursuing her own research, defying doctor's recommendations, finding the only doctor miles from New York City who would do a lumpectomy, and using vitamin drips that are still way beyond what most doctors know, care, or advise. And Deena did all this backwards and in high heels: a struggling single mother raising a young son while running a popular Upper West Side pottery studio and school, back when the neighborhood was grubby, dodgy, and cheap. She was a double pioneer as a woman entrepreneur and—somewhat less glamorous—a bold, prescient cancer patient.

I always knew that if it *came to this*—another euphemism—Deena would be my guru. Coach-like, methodical, and unafraid of bad news, she projected an exterior of calm, whatever was crackling underneath. I knew she would be an antidote to my own high anxiety and that of my sister and two women I talk to frequently, Zanti and Evelyn, who both had close family and friends who had recently died of cancer, and who both assured me that *everything is going to be fine* rather than entertaining the possibility that it wouldn't be.

From the first phone call, Deena skipped the niceties, skipped what Joan Didion, in her novel *Run, River* calls "the comfortable, loving fictions," and went straight to: "This is what you do next."

"Take James to your appointments and tell him to bring a notebook. Go with a list of questions. Tell him to write down everything because even if you think you'll remember, you won't. Ask questions even when the doctors are sick of answering them. Get all the information before making any decisions."

"When I went through this myself," I'd heard her say many times over the years, to me and those she counseled through cancer, "I thought of what I was doing—grilling the doctors, doing the research—as a job. It saved my life and kept me from feeling powerless."

Jumping

Power. Is it something we only think about when we lose ours or don't have it to begin with? Like good health itself, more noticed when it threatens to leave than when it's there every day, not getting in anyone's way. When my fingers felt the lump, my personal power—my sense that I am more or less in control of my life—collapsed instantaneously, a puppet with its strings cut. The only thing that restored that feeling, however chimerical, however brief, was taking action, even making a phone call. As long as I was doing something, doing anything, to gather information or coax my lymph node to shrink, I was OK. More or less.

Another find on Google's lists of natural remedies was worth a shot: jumping jacks. Off I went that weekend to my health club yoga studio in the empty off hours and jumped. And jumped. And jumped some more.

I was like a naked woman running out of a burning building, beyond self-consciousness as I jumped up and down, waving my arms, hundreds of times. The effort reminded me of a teenage remedy for getting rid of unwanted pregnancies, jumping repeatedly from the bathtub ledge to the floor—and was probably as effective. But like the desperate teenager, I jumped until my knees ached. On my way home, I stopped at a Jamba Juice shop I had never entered and combed the menu for cures. I knocked back two shots of wretched forest green wheat grass juice with turmeric, seven dollars each, because it was said to . . . what was it exactly? Reduce inflammation? Boost my immune system?

I was going to outsmart this little fucker in my arm in record time and then get on with the rest of my life. Seven dollars a pop? Or was it two for seven? I would have shelled out twice as much.

What I Do for Money

Speaking of spending money, which is connected at the hip to making money. Which is connected in the US to health, healthcare, health insurance, and, especially if you are a person like I am without a salary, to the slippery downward slope toward the P-words: penury and poverty. And a person like I am whose money-making is a seasonal endeavor. Adding to my anxiety about the lump was the fact that the next three months were always the busiest and most lucrative of my annual calendar, beginning with three weeks of preparing and then teaching a fiction workshop, followed by many months when I would make the money to buy double shots of wheat grass juice and health insurance that was almost two grand a month.

I was already engaged in the logistics and mechanics of illness, even before it was a reality. When playwright Eve Ensler learned she had uterine cancer that had spread to other organs, she was on her way to Congo to open a woman's shelter. At a slightly different point in my own drama, I was on my way to . . . my living room to prepare for a fiction workshop that I teach at the New York State Summer Writers Institute, at Skidmore College. I had stacks of reading and weeks of preparation, along with tending a group of high school students I tutor privately on their college applications. These are sources of income as well as deep connections I have with many dozens of people for six months of the year, every year. We talk about books, writers, words and sentences on the page, and the ambitions and motivations behind them. In the interstices, we sometimes talk about more personal matters. This is another way of saying that if I'm not writing my own work, I am helping other people write theirs. Another way of saying that the period from June to December is the worst possible time to come down with . . . whatever this was.

James and I were leaving for Saratoga Springs on July 2. And I would know Monday June 13, when I went to the radiology lab, what this lump was. Until then, I was swilling all the turmeric tea and apple cider vinegar I could stand. And jumping up and down like a maniac.

The Scan Man

A narrow, windowless room with beige walls, low lighting, a sonogram screen at my head, and James perched at the foot of the table. The technician snapped pictures and pressed a wand into the bulge as I raised my right arm above my head. She took ten or twelve shots, left the room, and returned with a doctor I'd encountered before. Small, wiry, not young, and possessed of an expressive face I came to wish was more stolid.

There are two lymph nodes, he said, squinting, hovering closer to the screen behind my head and to the right.

Two? How did I only feel one?

"The second is underneath the first," he explained. "How do you feel?" He did not step away from the screen.

"Fine. I had a physical two weeks ago. Everything was normal except a very elevated parathyroid hormone level which I've had for more than twenty years."

The parathyroid, a tiny gland behind the thyroid, controls the bones' ability to absorb calcium. When calcium courses through the bloodstream without being absorbed, it usually causes intense, ongoing fatigue, a condition easily corrected with surgery. But my calcium levels were never so high that they caused fatigue, and over the years, several doctors had advised against the operation. Over time, the results are osteoporosis.

"Is there any cancer in your family?"

"My father had lung cancer from smoking. When he was seventy-five."

"Did you cut your arm shaving recently?"

"No."

"Do you have a sore throat, anything like that?"

"I had a bit of a cold a week ago. It's gone now."

He told the technician to wand the edge of my right breast and then my other armpit. "I don't see anything there that concerns me," he said, studying the screen. "Well . . . If it doesn't go away, come back in a few weeks. At that point, I'd recommend a biopsy or a PET scan."

"Do you think it's lymphoma?" I got up the gumption to ask. I didn't tell him that two years before, I'd gotten the ends of my fingers covered with Krazy Glue while repairing a piece of pottery, and, in a panic, had soaked them in bleach to get the Krazy Glue off. It was the fingers of my right hand, and here was the lump, in my right armpit.

"Not from what we know now," he said.

He did not exactly tap dance out of the room, but because I felt fine and because there was little random cancer in my family—and because I didn't yet know how to translate these doctor messages—I left feeling buoyed. These lumps could well disappear with a few more mugs of turmeric tea. In the lobby of the clinic, we ran into the doctor again, and I said to James, with the doctor close by, "You see why I love these people? They tell you everything right here. You don't have to wait."

The doctor, a radiologist with many miles on his odometer, smiled in a kindly but concerned way, a pinched smile, which I noted but chose to read as more cheerful than it might have been. Yet seeing him again made me feel better, and the best news was that no one was panicking. They wanted me back in a few weeks. I knew that if they saw so much as a dot on your breast X-ray, they did not tell you to come back in three weeks. And I was confident that enough turmeric tea and a daily shot of wheat grass would shrink this thing—these things—before my next encounter with destiny.

Chocolate Babka

For the birds. My parents' all-purpose expression for something or someone not performing well. *That movie—that doctor—that restaurant—was for the birds.* While I waited for the lumps to shrink, I read student short stories, worked on Skype with the high school kids I tutored, and wrote the introduction I would give at the writers' conference, but my concentration was for the birds. I would read two or three paragraphs before I realized I hadn't been paying attention and start over. I'd vow to focus, but by the end of the page, I'd gotten ten percent of it. It felt like slipping on ice every time I stood up and took a few steps. And every fifteen or twenty minutes, I touched the lump in my armpit.

Maybe a bit smaller? And why was it so difficult to get a sense of? It moved around and sometimes it felt round and other times ovoid, and *it was not going away*. But it had to be getting smaller, with the barrage of remedies taking aim at it. And I had to concentrate. I had gotten through four of the nine short stories. I could do this. Of course I could. But between the lines of the text, I kept seeing flashes of Sue Briskman in the senior lounge in her white ribbed turtleneck, then Sue in her coffin, which thank God had been closed. Out of sight for forty years, forty-five years, she was back with a vengeance.

Anxiety had killed my appetite. I was losing weight, which was kind of fun and kind of scary. Wasn't unexplained weight loss one of the Seven Warning Signs of cancer? But wait! It *was* explained. I had another of the warning signs: *a thickening or lump in the breast or elsewhere*. How many boxes on the list did I need to check off in order to win the prize? I shoved a few hardboiled eggs down my throat in the morning with coffee, but I had to find something with more calories to keep me going. Even when my insides groaned with longing for calories, there was nothing in the apartment I wanted to consume.

I wandered four blocks over to Zabar's in search of high-end comfort food. With no destination in mind, I passed three hundred kinds of cheese from France and Holland and Brooklyn and a case of petit fours, cupcakes, and pear tarts and a refrigerated case of smoked salmon and white fish. When I stopped at a set of shelves packed with loaves of babka, alternating chocolate and cinnamon, my brakes went on. Babka was the right mix of sweet, complicated, and forbidden, the brioche-like braided bread laced with chocolate so nutritionally useless I might as well guzzle cane sugar straight from the box. That day I could trick myself into thinking it had medicinal properties.

At home, after twenty seconds in the microwave, the huge chunk of cake went limp, and the dark chocolate oozed like peanut butter.

When I stopped before the piece was gone, it was to cut off another hunk and zap it while I returned to slice number one—like someone lighting a cigarette while they're still smoking one. As I stood at the kitchen counter, most of the loaf disappeared down my gullet in fifteen minutes.

Had this been the best idea I'd had in a long time or the worst? I had not touched the lump in my arm or *even thought about it* for half an hour! But a wave of sugar fatigue hit me, and I stumbled across the apartment to lie down as a text came through.

James: "Anything you want from Zabar's?"

Me (do I confess now or wait until he's back?): "The usual?"

That meant a few pieces of grilled chicken and grilled salmon and some containers of roasted vegetables. Would I hide the incriminating piece of babka that was left—evidence of my addled state of mind—or would I show it to him? I didn't want him to know quite how out of control my anxiety was, but how long could I keep it a secret? Or maybe it wasn't a secret. Even without my broadcasting it every minute, I was probably a dead giveaway. James would understand—of course he would!—that this was just a phase I was going through, like a pregnant woman. Or a woman waiting to find out if she has cancer.

Nam Myoho Renge Kyo

"Try chanting," implored my sister Nancy, my only sister, my only sibling. "It's great for anxiety. Please."

I was worried about cancer, and she was worried about my anxiety.

Tibetan Buddhist chanting has helped her through all kinds of spiritual and psychic crises, places where psychotherapy doesn't go. *Nam Myoho Renge Kyo*. It was that simple, she explained, and you just say it over and over until calm descends on you like soft rain.

"Try it," she said. "I'll send you chanting beads and a booklet. I'd come to the city myself"—she lives in New Jersey—"but I have friends who live near you, and they'll come in a flash and chant with you. It's very soothing because whatever's wrong with you, the *anxiety is not helping.*"

"I think I'll pass," I said. "But thank you."

Or maybe I didn't say thank you. I was distracted. The truth was that even in what felt like my darkest hour to date, I still had no team spirit, a quality or anti-quality I'd identified with decades before while reading Muriel Spark's novel *The Prime of Miss Jean Brodie*. Florence Nightingale, Miss Brodie opined to her high school girls, had no team spirit. Nor did Helen of Troy, Cleopatra, or the Queen of England. I was no more interested in chanting with people I didn't know than I had been in joining the Brownies or the Girl Scouts as a kid, in being on a sports team, or going to work in an office every day. And the problem, the actual problem, was not my anxiety.

Despite my reluctance, when Nancy came to visit me, she said, "Let's chant."

"Now?"

"Now." I looked from her to her husband to James, all of us sitting quietly in the living room, the specter of my having cancer the only subject on any of our minds. "Repeat after me," Nancy said, closed her eyes, and intoned, *"Nam Myoho Renge Kyo,"* over and over until the rest of us got the hang of it and followed along, stumbling some but chanting, the two sisters and the two husbands, willing, as people are when the backdrop of good health goes dark, to do just about anything that might allay our fears and recast the storyline.

We must have chanted the phrase—and who knew or cared what it meant?—thirty or forty times before I realized that it was having no effect on me. I cracked open my eyes and was touched to see everyone else, eyes closed, burbling these syllables, and to see my sister across the living room, her hands delicately on her thighs, leading us. But where? She looked peaceful but determined. And I understood that this was about calming her nerves as much as mine, maybe more than mine. It gave her something to do besides worry that I might die. But it wasn't having the same effect on me.

A short time later, James and I visited her for the weekend, and the first thing she did was take me to her friend's house for more chanting. In the vast suburban living room was an elaborate Buddhist altar the size of a home entertainment center that briefly made me ashamed of my skepticism. This worked for them—why not me? I hadn't wanted to be a Girl Scout when I was eight, but I didn't need to be churlish now, did I? I would give it another chance, until I heard we would be there for *an hour*. I quietly told Nancy I wouldn't last. I was open to this but only to—let's call it—drive-by chanting. *Nam Myoho Renge Kyo*. Fifteen minutes on the outside. And even that . . .

I tried to give myself over to it—the voices, the rhythms, Nancy's kindness and her friend's, the enveloping altar—while I marveled at Nancy's discipline and her singing of another Tibetan chant that was five or six dense pages of syllables that changed from line to line and that she chanted without a hiccup.

Back in the city when the weekend was over, she phoned to see how I was doing.

"The same," I said. I was a chanting flop, not quite a chanting denier but just impervious to its charms and wonders.

"What about Cymbalta again?" she suggested, knowing that the antidepressant I'd taken for a few brief periods, in smaller doses, also relieves anxiety. I had an unfinished bottle in the drawer of my night-stand.

"Excellent idea."

"How long before they kick in?"

"Ten days, two weeks."

"Maybe the lymph node will have shrunk by then," Nancy said brightly.

The node will shrink. The node will shrink. The node will shrink.

That was a chant I could get behind, but my hand slipped easily into the drawer by my bed, and I twisted off the childproof lid and counted how many pills I had left.

Comfortable Loving Fictions

I began every day with a ritual: walking to the living room and sitting down cross-legged on the thick rug so I could feel around for the lump. It was hard to find while lying in bed; in many positions, it was gone, hiding somewhere in the shoulder girdle. Sitting on the floor, I could find it more easily. Some mornings I couldn't find it, and for five or ten minutes, I would be my happy former self—but happier and even more grateful than before because I had come so close to the abyss. But when I poked around some more, there it *always always always* was. But smaller. Most definitely smaller.

"I think you're going to be fine," James said on a regular basis be-cause I didn't need to be mainlining babka for him to see I was not myself.

"And you think that because?"

"You've got energy. Color in your face. There's nothing sickly about you."

I thought again of the Joan Didion line from *Run, River*. You can tell or you can be told "the comfortable loving fictions," the ones James was telling me, and the ones Zanti and Evelyn patiently repeated in a rainbow of variations: "Lymph nodes take a while to shrink." "Give it time." "You're fine." "If this were cancer, you'd have other symptoms."

Never mind that a lump in a place where it's not supposed to be is a symptom. Yet as rattled as I was by the bump and the waiting, I felt an obligation to James and our relationship to not devolve openly into the hot, heaping mess that I was. When he came home in the late afternoons and we swapped stories of our time apart, I told him about my medical discoveries for the day, which I delivered with the upbeat energy I conveyed in my usual reports. "You know what I learned today?" I might begin brightly. "I've been reading about wheat grass juice, and it looks like if I drink two shots a day with turmeric and ginger, that'll give me enough antioxidants to cure a horse." Or was it a chipmunk? My first husband was intermittently depressed and could easily slip into gloom and sadness. James was an eternal—infuriating—optimist, but I was beginning to see that this might have its practical value.

James' refusal to swim in my pool of terror kept me close to the surface and made it possible to do the work I needed to do: read a stack of student short stories, prepare my class syllabus, and engage on Skype coaching sessions with three, four, sometimes five high school students a day on their college essays. I never mentioned my state of mind or my situation to them or their parents, until a mother called whose daughter I had worked with the year before. The mom was a radiologist, and the year before, she had confided some of her own difficulties to me, so when she asked how I was, I did not break down, but I broke my vow of silence.

"I have a lump in my armpit," I admitted. "I had a sonogram ten days ago."

I did not want to share any news with parents that would make them question my long-term fitness to help their children as they prepared college applications for the November 1 and the January 1 deadlines. Their anxiety about their children's futures was on a par with my own about my health. This too was pressing on me: if this lump was the dreaded thing, how would I carry on with my work? What would I say to parents—and when? Could their already-frayed nerves take another uncertainty? *The woman we hired to help our kid get into college has a fatal illness.* This did not have a good ring to it.

"How big is it?" the radiologist mom asked.

I found the report from the lab and read the numbers out to her:

"The larger one is 1.9 x 1.2 x 1.1 cm. The other one is 1.7 x 0.8 cm."

"That sounds good," she said. "It's when they're three centimeters or bigger that you have to worry."

What a relief. And what a good idea it had been to confide in her!

I was certain that if I kept up my natural remedies regimen—the tea, the jumping jacks, and the steam room I had added—the evidence would wither away. Not everyone was as vigilant and disciplined as I was, despite another loaf of babka that I decorously stopped short of finishing. My exemplary behavior and self-control would be rewarded. Of course it would. Everyone said so. But five days later, having read eight of the nine student short stories, and ten days before I was to leave for my teaching gig, I could no longer tell anyone who asked me that I felt fine.

The Thing about Illness . . .

Even the threat of an illness before it has a name—it pulverizes the routines and expectations of ordinary life. Suddenly taking out the trash is tinged with meaning, the anticipation of loss. Or is it me? Is this Roz Chast-level obsession only because I don't have a nine-to-five job or a family to support? It's only when I work with students that I can shut off the terror machine. My brain is not capable of multitasking: when I give the kids my attention, I've got no room for the symphony of existential dread. When I'm done with them, I have plenty of time in which to wonder whether it's good luck or bad luck that I am self-employed and have no one's bills to pay but my own, which leaves me free to wallow in free-floating fear.

But even my fear, which is as heavy and graceless as an anvil, does not keep me from acknowledging intense feelings of gratitude throughout the day. The evidence is all around me that I am rich in friends and rich in love but dirt poor in emotional shock absorbers.

Some of the people I am closest to know that I'm waiting for answers, but we have not told Emily. "Should we tell her?" I ask James one of those nights when I'm taking a weird delight in feeling my unusually svelte hip-bones through my filmy summer nightgown. How much more weight would I lose just from being anxious, and how much would be too much?

"Let's wait until we find out what's going on," he says kindly.

Of course that's his answer. If I were thinking clearly, I would not have had to ask.

Spaghetti and Meatballs

At five o'clock on the morning of June 25, I woke up with burning in my armpits and burning that radiated through my upper chest.

Sylvie the NP was not in at 9:00 a.m., and I was put through to one of the doctors, who could see details of my recent visit on the computer. "I think I need to be in the hospital," I said. "There is something *very wrong* with me." When I explained my symptoms, the doctor was mystified. "And the swollen lymph nodes are still there."

"I think you need to be patient," she said. "Lymph nodes sometimes take a month to go down. Your blood work was fine when you saw Sylvie two weeks ago, except for the elevated parathyroid levels. Maybe that's causing some of the discomfort."

"I feel *terrible*."

Didn't it count for something that I rarely called the doctor for anything and never to declare that I felt *terrible*? I will cop to being a hypochondriac, but never one who called a doctor and said, "I need to be in the hospital." I had been a hospital patient for exactly one night in my entire life.

"You're very anxious," she said. "And I'm sure that's contributing to your overall health. I'm sure you're just fighting off an infection."

This wasn't happening, was it? In the year 2017, a woman doctor in an office of women doctors is telling me the problem is my anxiety?

"I'm not faking this," I said. "Something is wrong with me."

"Why don't you come in and do some more blood work? It should set your mind at ease. I'll connect to you the front desk so you can make an appointment with Sylvie. She'll be back in two days."

My chest burned, and when I stood up, I was unsteady on my feet. My two cups of coffee didn't give me half the energy I usually had. By noon, my legs felt leaden. Mystery had seeped into every waking moment: the mystery of whether I had a fatal illness, whether I could finish preparing for my class, and whether I'd have the strength to teach on a college campus in nine days—schlepping back and forth across the quadrangle four times a day—when I could barely cross my living room.

The following day, I called the director of the writers' workshop and explained I had an assortment of ailments—sticking with fatigue and elevated parathyroid, not the lump—and told him I was afraid I might not be up to teaching.

"Don't think twice about it. Take care of yourself. I have someone I can ask to fill in. The most important thing is that you're not gravely ill."

Well, actually . . . I had buried the lede when talking to him. No need to go all the way to cancer and freak people out when I had another medical problem nowhere near as unsettling—and maybe the intense fatigue was my parathyroid finally kicking into high gear as it never had.

I lay back on the couch, the only direction I could move, and closed my eyes against the intense midday sun, against the view of the Hudson River and New Jersey from my windows. The weight of the teaching was gone. The fear I'd flub the week was over, but as my fingers drifted to their familiar place in the hinge of my arm and the thing— The Thing from Outer Space—was still there, my insides clenched with an airplane turbulence intensity: This plane might really be going down.

Why was it taking so long for this drama to resolve? The lump was right there! I could feel it all the time. I *did* feel it all the time. James watched me feeling it all the time. It was as obvious as a plate of spaghetti and meatballs.

A Breast Specialist?

How long had it been by then? Three weeks? Almost time for another visit to the radiology lab. And much too soon to call the former head of Memorial Sloan Kettering. That was an emergency number, like breaking the glass box to call the fire department. But I called a psychiatrist friend who ran a department in a major hospital and whose practice was more medicine than talk therapy. I said I thought I had lymphoma.

"Liz, don't catastrophize," he said kindly. "Do you have night sweats?"

"No."

"That's good. Any other medical issues?"

"Elevated parathyroid levels—much higher than usual."

"The symptoms from that are global—fatigue especially."

"I should be getting a biopsy or a PET scan soon," I told my friend. But when I wrote to Sylvie the following day through the patient portal, asking for a referral to get either procedure, as the radiologist suggested, she refused.

"I would recommend a repeat sonogram rather than a PET Scan. . . . Sonogram is a less expensive and less invasive test. The radiologist recommended follow-up examination, and if persisting then additional work-up. I would re-examine with sonogram to let us know what the next best steps are. . . . Your anxiety surrounding this matter is intense, and therefore we should take further steps for reassurance or expediency pending results."

I was livid at her refusal and at her reason—*sonogram is less expensive?!*—and at her obliviousness to the psychic and physical costs of making this drag on even longer. I had already canceled one summer activity and one source of income. We were days from July, when I had plans to go away in the middle of the month for three weeks, and when doctors routinely take vacations too. How much more uncertainty could I endure when a biopsy or a PET scan would settle it? I had just begun paying $1,800 a month for health insurance that would start July 1, and it was not to cut corners on tests.

I went over her head and scheduled a phone appointment with the doctor who owned the practice and was the doctor of record on insurance forms. On the phone that evening, she was brusque, insisting the lump was a "reactive lymph node" that would soon go down—reacting, that is, to a nearby infection—and uninterested in doing anything more aggressive than waiting. She later sent a message through the patient portal: "If it would help your anxiety, do you want to see a breast specialist?"

If it would help your anxiety?

Since when had I moved to Freud's Vienna, land of hysterical women who needed their inexplicable anxieties muffled? I was so enraged by her out-of-left-field suggestion—what was a breast specialist anyway?—that I didn't answer. I fumed. I called a friend who was also her patient, and she fumed with me. This frosty, difficult-to-reach doctor was the gatekeeper, and I didn't have the medical chops to challenge her. But I knew I did not need a breast specialist.

Plenty of Time

Not long after, Sylvie invited me to the office for another round of blood work, to placate my anxiety, and so I could pick up the referral for the next sonogram. When I described my ongoing fatigue and the mysterious burning in the upper chest, Sylvie suggested I see an endocrinologist about my elevated parathyroid. That at least responded to some of my symptoms.

As she handed me the two referrals, she said, "I'm one of the most conservative and conscientious people in this office. Another sonogram will tell us if we need to do any more. And it will give us plenty of time to do it. And it will go a long way toward alleviating your anxiety."

Plenty of time? New York was about to become a medical ghost town. And why was my anxiety the issue? My lymph node was the size of a walnut. If they find a lentil-size lump in someone's breast, it's a code blue emergency. They biopsy it before sundown.

Sylvie smiled warmly—a practiced smile, a professional gesture—as I swung the straps of my purse over my shoulder to leave. I smiled back—a sort of smile, pinched, insincere, enraged. But as I stepped out of the office, I could feel my rage dissolve into relief.

I remembered my sister's one-liner about life in New York, which encapsulates our growing up with an angry father in an angry city: "Excuse me, sir, do you happen to know the time, or should I just go fuck myself right now?" I am usually good at defending myself when I feel mistreated, but I didn't insist on a biopsy or a PET scan because, as much as I wanted an answer, I was relieved there would be another pause in facing what I was beginning to believe was the truth. And if

I had known anything at all about biopsies, I would have insisted on an FNA, which means Fine Needle Aspiration, and all it requires is a needle and a microscope. It can't diagnose anything, but it detects the presence of abnormal cells in minutes.

My new expensive insurance would begin on July 1. I would not need referrals from Sylvie to see any doctor I pleased, but I still would not be able to order my own biopsy. In the meantime, my New Yorker moxie had vanished.

Daughters

Emily has been in my life for two decades, for so long that I could easily say *I'm used to her*, but that is not quite true. She stays in our New York apartment often when she comes to the city for rehearsals and performances. We hear her practicing the violin behind a closed door and see her come in wiped out after ten hours of rehearsals and late at night after concerts. I know well the routines and rigors of her life, but when I see her play on stage or on a video, I'm transfixed by what she does, by the talent and skill and sheer work it takes to dance as she does across the strings, the tightrope, of a violin.

When I tell her sometimes, "You have the hardest job in New York," she makes light of it. "You always say that," she says, which I think means that she thinks that I don't get how many other people do what she does. I must sound to her like a gloating parent who thinks everything her kid does is a work of genius. Perhaps I should amend my statement: violinists—all of them—have the hardest job in New York, and one of them happens to be in my apartment. Brain surgeons at least have teams of associates. Writers—well, I can get up a hundred times a day from my computer and still do my job.

I am not quite used to her talent yet, or maybe I will always be in awe of it because that's the nature of such gifts. I know that when I hear her talking about music with James, with all of their verve and precision, their private language, it's a connection I will never have with either of them, and I'm enchanted all over again. Startled anew that these otherworldly beings found their way into my prosaic life in the last year of the twentieth century—and that they are still here. That we are all still here. That my divorce from my first husband eventually led us here. On her birthday cards, I have written that the years since she and her father entered my life have been the happiest of my life.

My first marriage was happy for many years, though at the heart of it was my husband's deep sadness at losing his son—and my own longing for a daughter I had wanted to adopt from Vietnam, where, long before I knew him, my husband had spent almost three years as a US diplomat during the war.

When I met James three years after my marriage ended, the soundtrack changed, the narrative brightened: I was rich in James and Emily. She is almost the same age as that distant daughter who got away. The child I did not go to Vietnam to bring back home with me because I got divorced instead.

Drop another pin in the place on the map marked Vietnam.

Do You Want to Talk About it?

I first read Susan Sontag's *Illness as Metaphor* in 1992, curious about it as a writer and still an inhabitant of the kingdom of the well. The landscape has changed dramatically since it was published in 1978, and since 1975, when Sontag was given a grim prognosis for her stage four breast cancer. Yet the book is still a touchstone, a learned investigation on a disease that's still baffling, still killing. She describes an idea, still prevalent at the time, of the "cancer personality," a psychological cause—repression—to explain why some got it and others didn't. It was magical thinking, hardly an idea Sontag herself subscribed to, but in the absence of greater understanding and effective treatment, it filled a void for many and answered the question "Why me?" Easy: Because you're uptight. You've repressed your feelings, especially your sexual feelings!

It was the era when expressing emotions as flamboyantly as possible was all the rage (see Primal Scream Therapy and John and Yoko's 1969 Bed-ins for Peace). Americans and some celebrities across the pond were committed to advancing the sexual revolution and freeing themselves from the shackles of puritanical mores. If you didn't get cancer, you could comfort yourself with the notion that you were not so repressed after all. And if you got it, you could remember a time or three when you held back letting rip your deepest feelings.

The message was that repression is so toxic it might actually cause this deadly disease. The famous Ed Koren *New Yorker* cartoon, c. 1975, of the mother saying to the child who's dropped his ice cream cone, "Do you want to talk about it?" was the cherry on top of the national obsession with exploring every feeling that came our way.

By 2017, when I found the lumps in my armpit, we knew better. We knew more about what's inherited and genetic, and what in the environment causes cancer—though we might have been better off thinking a certain personality type was the culprit, because the answer is that nearly everything causes it: nicotine, the sun, relatives with cancer, obesity, burnt meat, advancing age, sitting too much, not exercising enough, the herbicide Roundup, chemicals in hair dye, cell phones (maybe), sugar (maybe), proximity to power stations, radiation, pesticides, preservatives, PCBs, perfluorooctanoic acid (PFOA, or C-8), and entire geographic regions where these chemicals were either manufactured or dumped, including Monsanto's plant in Nitro, West Virginia, where Agent Orange was made from the 1940s to the 1970s, and Parkersburg, West Virginia, where Dupont's plants leaked PFOA into the water. The company eventually settled more than three thousand personal injury claims associated with six diseases, including kidney and testicular cancers.

In the twenty-first century, the reputed cause of cancer has morphed from cancer personality to cancer-inviting behavior: smoking, suntanning, eating some of the foods listed in the USDA's four basic food groups list, and neglecting routine colonoscopies and mammograms. In the good news column, the twenty-first century has given scientists the ability to quantify what percentage of new cancers are "potentially avoidable"—42 percent! This includes "19 percent caused by smoking and the 18 percent that are caused by a combination of excess body weight, physical inactivity, excess alcohol consumption, and poor nutrition." The precision of the 42 percent means that 58 percent of cancers are "unavoidable." With the right assortment of behaviors, you might dodge the "potentially avoid-ables," but you are just as susceptible as everyone else to those that are "unavoidable." And "unavoidable" is a euphemism for, "We have no blinking idea why you got this."

Our Bodies Are Disasters Waiting to Happen

Now that we're past the Cancer Personality Nonsense, it's understood that we're playing a game of Russian Roulette Without End, whether we want to play or not. One in two women will be struck with cancer (and one in eight with breast cancer) and one in three men (one in 883 of them with breast cancer). Yet with all this sickness in our midst, it's curious that hypochondria—acute worry over illness and the pos-sibilities of illness—only officially afflicts five percent of the popula-tion, and that, according to Wikipedia, the most famous hypochon-driacs have been men. And men you'd imagine who had more pressing matters to worry about, including James Boswell, Charles Darwin, Marcel Proust, Leonard Bernstein, Andy Warhol, and Woody Allen.

Who, I wondered, are the famous women hypochondriacs? Flor-ence Nightingale is the only historic name that one Wikipedia page spits up. But the facts suggest that she was bedridden for so long be-cause she really *was* quite ill—with symptoms resembling chronic fa-tigue—after spending two years tending British soldiers in and around Turkey during the Crimean War. How could it be that poor, noble Florence, who practically invented modern nursing, is the only nota-ble woman extreme worrier about her health? So much serious illness comes our way, but only one woman represents us across the centuries? On another day, I find another Wikipedia list of hypochondriacs in history—and the only woman's name is Jiang Qing, also known as Madame Mao. If we go farther afield and search "hysteria" and "depression," women are amply represented, but hypochondria itself appears to be a male-dominated obsession. How can that be?

Once I put my mind to this query, I came up with a theory of the case. It's not that we don't worry, and worry acutely—God knows!—but that *all* of us worry, with varying degrees of intensity, because we have so many body parts to worry about, and they are all—we learn soon enough—disasters waiting to happen. How could historians choose a half dozen famous women who worry more than the rest of us worry? Our worrying is so deep and widespread that it used to have a raft of alarming names, including hysteria, madness, and neurasthenia. These days, when we do express concern about medical matters, they are too often trivialized as "psychosomatic" or stemming from anxiety. And some have argued that conditions that affect more women than men, notably chronic fatigue and fibromyalgia, are studied less rigorously than illnesses more common in men.

Despite ongoing controversies around the differences between the brains of men and women, there's little dispute about the huge, persistent gender gap between men's and women's well-being in every metric of physical and mental health. Are the differences nature, nurture, or a combination we will never be able to isolate and measure? Whatever the origins, there is no getting around the facts: men suffer more heart disease, kidney stones, hernia, gout, and alcoholism than women do, and they die on average five years before women do. But women are much more likely to report—and seek treatment for—their higher levels of stress, depression, and anxiety. (A wild thought: we're more stressed and anxious because men refuse to take better care of themselves?)

Leaving aside strife between the sexes, it's a hard fact that women have what to worry about from an early age. And as we look around at our mothers and elders, we hear about their medical worries even before those worries land on us. But whether we've paid any mind to our mother's worries and problems, it sure gets our attention when we begin to bleed profusely every month. When we learn the gravity of what it means. When we discover that even if a partner shares contraceptive considerations, it's the woman who waits every month for her period. And these worries are merely when we're in perfectly good health—before we learn that our breasts are actually bullseyes, deadly targets waiting to be hit, not to mention the vulnerability of the entire reproductive tract. If we have children, we transfer our vigilance to them and their bodies. Once we're too old to get pregnant, when our bodies creak and rumble in reverse, we've still got the monthly self-exams, the yearly mammograms, the tumors that might pop up in all the hidden places.

It's unusual for men to hyper-focus on their bodies, on everything that might go wrong, because not as many parts break down as regularly, and men are less inclined to notice if they do. Study after study confirms that they go less often to fewer doctors and pay less attention to symptoms than women do. When they fret to worrisome degrees, they get a label slapped on them—hypochondriac!—and sometimes an entry in Wikipedia. *Poor guys! So worried something might go wrong!* A friend lived in an apartment building with a screening room where, she told me, Woody Allan invited friends to see his latest movies, and he held a separate screening just for his doctors.

I come to see that worrying about our bodies and our health—and that of our children and spouses—is just women being women. It's as natural as brushing our hair, once we learn the costs of not brushing it.

"To be born a woman is to know," wrote W. B. Yeats in "Adam's Curse," "although they do not talk of it at school—that we must labour to be beautiful."

And to be born a woman is to know that our bodies and especially our female parts are disasters waiting to happen. We don't have much of a choice but to deal with it, daily, weekly, monthly.

Even still, some of us worry more than others.

On Not Having Children

When people ask me if I have children, I mention Emily, but of course I did not raise her from birth—she was twelve when we met. Which gives me the room to wonder whether having had a child of my own might have moved me past some of my hypochondria. Might motherhood have toughened me up—having to confront someone else's frailties on a continuous basis, rather than just my own? And more significant but related: might it have made me less self-involved, less fascinated by my feelings, by the particulars of my past, the ghost of Sue Briskman, the *mishigas* of my family? It would certainly have given me another cast of characters and dramas to dwell among. Or would I have done what parents do and just passed on my own anxieties, delivered them to my kids in the same or slightly different containers?

Are our nervous systems heritable traits like the color of our eyes, the shape of our fingers? Did one of the traumas that plagued my mother's life—the infamous Hartford "Mad Dog Taborsky" murder of her brother—become part of her brain chemistry and thus part of mine? Or was his murder-by-handgun two months before my parents' wedding in 1950 just a sad story that was passed on to me as a child and that I investigated as an adult? I don't remember her having been excessively worried about her own health or mine, not more than an ordinary mother, but I remember the stories of Lou's murder in a hold-up in his liquor store, the wife and young daughters he left behind, the other Taborsky murders that followed, the trials, the publicity. The stories and her sorrow had a life of their own in our family that must have colored my sense of the fragility of things—and that Sue Briskman's random death might have intensified. But can these influences ever be untangled so precisely that we can say, "This fear comes from here and that fear from there"? Will neuroscience ever be able to identify what event caused which behavior? Which childhood trauma caused which adult phobia? Probably not.

But it seems reasonable to wonder how much these family stories played into my decision not to have a child when I was on the verge of moving ahead with an adoption. Or did my reluctance have more to do with the unhappy marriage I was in? Or was it my writerly ambitions? Growing up, I learned that women writers were childless: Jane Austen, the Brontës, George Eliot, Virginia Woolf. In the 1980s, when I began to publish, many women writers had only one child, the only number that such a fragile ecosystem—the combination of mother/writer/wife/and often breadwinner and writing professor—could support. There were exceptions, but Erica Jong, Alice Walker, Margaret Atwood, Joan Didion, Katha Pollitt, Alice Randall, Mary Morris, and Siri Hustvedt come to mind in the onesies category. I was deeply ambivalent about having a child myself, fearing an ecosystem imbalance, terrified I would never have enough time or money to do the child and the writing justice—and I'd mess them both up. And afraid of something else too: that the intensity of my love for a child would be too much to bear, and that my fear of losing this person might overwhelm me.

Although many male writers in these generations—Philip Roth, Don DeLillo, Jonathan Franzen, Junot Diaz—did not have kids, I'm taking a wild guess that the angst involved in their decisions rarely reached the levels of intensity that their female counterparts endured. In his *Paris Review* interview, George Saunders, who has two grown daughters, answers a direct, difficult question on the matter: "Do you think you'd be a different writer if you hadn't had children?"

> I'm not sure I would have ever published anything. Before we had our kids, I was a decent person, kind of habitually, but nothing felt morally urgent. Then the kids came, and everything suddenly mattered. The world had a moral edge. If I love these guys so much, it stands to reason that every other person in the world has somebody who loves them just as much—or they *should have* someone who loves them as much. The world was full of consequence. . . . It made work meaningful. I had a job as a tech writer, and it was a hard job, a combination of dull and demanding. Not exactly the life I'd dreamed of. And yet suddenly, it was an interesting place to write about, full, as it was, of people who had once been somebody's kids and were

often there for the same reason I was, to provide for their families.

I know other writers might feel that kids would impede them. And, depending on how you're wired and so on, that can definitely be true. But for me, it lit the world right up. And in the stories, you can see that. If a character of mine is insufficiently motivated, I just . . . give him a kid. Suddenly, they're not working that stupid job for themselves.

Kids opened up Saunders' emotional toolkit, waking his quiescent instincts. He could see that kids make lives matter in ways that they might not otherwise. They ramp the stakes up sky high. He doesn't mention the fear he feels as a parent, but when I read the tenderest scenes in *Lincoln in the Bardo*—the story of the death of Lincoln's young son—I imagine that he could not have written them without knowing what it means to fear losing a child.

Would you be a different writer if your life had been completely different?

Would you *be* a writer if your life had been completely different?

Roads taken, not taken, and lives cut short, like my mother's brother's. Lives survived, declined, imagined, envied, happily avoided, ardently longed for. Writing fiction is a way to dwell in these imaginary places.

My Own Private Hypochondria

My health phobias never took the form of hiding out in bed or frequent calls or visits to doctors. Except for routine visits and tests, I mostly avoided them. When I had problems, I researched "natural remedies" online, and they have often worked. When I've needed a person to talk to, I've called my sister or my friend Zanti, who both toil in the land of the body but think beyond the Conventional Western Medicine Seal of Approval. Nancy is a physical therapist who is certified in Feldenkrais, Zanti, an acupuncturist who has treated many seriously sick people over the decades. Between natural remedies and these two women, I've managed years of physical pain without drugs or surgery, and a few other minor ailments without purple reflux pills or prescription medication. Between them, they've answered my questions, settled my anxieties, and/or told me when it's time to see a doctor.

I don't remember every phone call to them over the years, but I remember with an embarrassing vividness how fragile and terrified I felt when I picked up the phone. It might only have been an ache or a spell of dizziness, but it was enough to activate my Sue-Briskman-nerve-center and most plaintive voice.

"That sounds completely normal," I hear my sister say or, "It's *nothing*. Really, *nothing!*" as she grows impatient with my anxiety. Zanti can hear the distress in my voice right away. "What is it, hon? What's wrong?"

And there is my fear of flying, which has been with me most of my adult life and which I've come to understand is a kind of hypochondria, nothing more or less than a fear of death. I fear it but I go places.

I pick seats in the back of the plane. I leave my will on the dining room table. I plan trips not quite believing that I will return home.

Jackie O's Hair

Shortly after Jackie Onassis died of lymphoma in 1994, I read in a magazine that she believed decades of coloring her hair black had brought it on. There were rumors after her death that there was a dip in requests for dark hair dye at some New York hair salons. Word was getting out—since confirmed in studies—that the darker the color and the more years you use permanent dyes, the more toxic it is.

The truth and history of hair dye is not a happy one—and not one that most media outlets want to publicize because hair care companies buy so much advertising, between shampoo, conditioner, and color. The existence of data that ordinary beauty products might cause The Dreaded One has created what seems to be a corporate conspiracy of silence that is wide and deep.

The American Cancer Society (ACS) has a webpage called simply "Hair Dyes," containing statement after statement that would probably shock most hairdressers and people who color their hair, starting with this:

> Researchers have been studying a possible link between hair dye use and cancer for many years. Studies have looked most closely at the risks of blood cancers (leukemias and lymphomas) and bladder cancer. While some studies have suggested possible links, others have not.

Following the equivocating "some studies do and some don't," the page breaks down the issue by types of dyes (semi-permanent and permanent are potentially most troublesome), types of cancers, types of studies (animals versus people), and the overall results of studies (mixed, which means some say yes), with bladder cancer a consistent issue for hairdressers but less so for customers. A separate sentence is devoted to breast cancer: "Many studies have not found an increase in risk, although some more recent studies have."

The page notes that the FDA does not regulate the ingredients in hair dyes—"thousands" of chemicals are involved—but does have guidelines about usage (don't get it near the eyes!) that suggest its toxicity. Notably, on the question of leukemias and lymphomas:

> Studies looking at a possible link between personal hair dye use and the risk of blood-related cancers such as leukemia and lymphoma have had mixed results. For example, some studies have found an increased risk of certain types of non-Hodgkin lymphoma (but not others) in women who use hair dyes, especially if they began use before 1980 and/or use darker colors. The same types of results have been found in some studies of leukemia risk. However, other studies have not found an increased risk. If there is an effect of hair dye use on blood-related cancers, it is likely to be small.

The advice section of the ACS website—"Should I limit my exposure to hair dyes?"—is far from a ringing endorsement of hair-dye safety. Nor does it mention the disquieting results of a major 2019 NIH study of 46,000 women that showed a slight increase in breast cancer for those who regularly use permanent hair dye and a more pronounced increase for Black women who regularly use permanent hair dye and/or chemical relaxers.

I suspect the failure of the study to gain traction in the media, despite an article about it in the *New York Times* and a three-minute piece on the *Today Show*, is evidence of a general denial: we don't want it to be true that our valiant efforts to look young may cause The Dreaded One. Compounding the unpleasantness of that possibility are all the advertising dollars that go into TV and print media. Furthermore, the mixed results of the studies—some say permanent dyes increase the chances of cancer and some say they don't—make scientists reluctant to issue definitive conclusions.

The result of these studies with mixed results is this milquetoast statement on the ACS website: "It's not clear how much personal hair dye use might raise cancer risk, if at all. Most studies done so far have not found a strong link, but more studies are needed to help clarify this issue." But the Jackie-O connection between blood cancer and dark hair dye was seared into my memory in 1995, and for a number of years, when I lived in Boston with James, I got my naturally dark brown locks colored at a salon in Cambridge that catered to cancer patients. I understood that the dye they used was less toxic than the ordinary kind, though now I am not so sure, since the job would have required the usual chemical culprits.

The chemical used for dark hair—the one of greatest concern—is para-phenylenediamine, or PPD, which is banned in hair dyes in France, Germany, and Sweden. The Environmental Working Group's (EWG) Skin Deep website, which rates ingredients in personal care products, rates PPD seven out of ten in toxicity. Maybe there *was* a secret ingredient in the Cambridge salon's dye, but I didn't know enough to ask for details. When I moved back to New York, I couldn't find another salon that used that supposedly less toxic product. My solution was to color my hair as infrequently as I could get away with. As a writer, I work at home, and my social life is among close friends, not people I am trying to impress with perfectly coifed and colored hair. Back then, I got my hair colored for special occasions or when it was Unbearable—whichever came first—but the dangers of it were always lurking, sometimes more noisily than others.

Nora, Mary, Susan

There was her photograph at the top of the bright white *Huffington Post* main page. Her radiant smile, her dark brown shaggy bob with a few reddish highlights. This powerful woman who had the world by a string—and beneath it her name in big letters and her dates: May 19, 1941–June 26, 2012.

Nora Ephron was dead, and when I tore through the text to find out the cause of death, I did a double take: myelodysplastic syndrome, a kind of leukemia. Another blood cancer. Another woman obsessed with her carefully coiffed dark brown hair. In one of the essays in *I Feel Bad About My Neck*, she writes that she got her hair "done" twice a week. She doesn't say *colored* twice a week—surely it wasn't. But no one that obsessed would skimp on the color the way I did.

In May 2015—another double-take when photographer Mary Ellen Mark, age seventy-five—who colored her hair jet black—succumbed to the same blood disease. Although Susan Sontag, who had famously dyed her hair black but for a dramatic shock of white at the front, had died in 2004, Mark's death reminded me that Sontag too had died of MDS, which she believed had been brought on by the cancer treatments she'd had decades before. As Nora lay in her hospital bed in the last month of her life, she read in horror about Sontag's MDS. Had any of them ever thought about hair dye as a culprit, or was this my own paranoid, hypochondriacal thinking?

Still, I kept dunking my scalp—while I diligently consumed organic food, drank organic milk, and avoided GORE-TEX, Teflon, and Scotchguard products because they sometimes still contained chemicals (PFOAs, PFAs) that made the products water repellent and possibly toxic when we're exposed to them over long periods.

When I learned that PFAs are used to make most dental flosses glide easily between teeth, I switched to organic floss, with some brands made of silk fibers and others of nylon. As an urban survivalist, I didn't fool around when it came to avoiding per- and polyfluoroalkyl substances in my mouth, my body, or my home, but the psychic cost of letting my hair grow out gray was, even for me, too high. I wasn't obsessed with fashion or beauty or the idea of "putting myself together," but a head of gray hair was a dirge too far. I might as well have worn a sign that said, "Next Stop: Old-age Home."

That changed in late 2014 when a new hairdresser who gave me a fantastic haircut messed up royally with the brown dye. When he was done, I could see the gray was gone, and I was in a rush to go to a birthday celebration. It was dark outside and dimly lit in the restaurant. The next morning, I stood at the bathroom mirror and discovered my hair was the unmistakable color of tar. Getting it back to brown would cost hundreds of dollars, take months of highlights, hours upon hours in the salon, my head covered like a Christmas tree with little squares of aluminum foil—a practice I had never indulged in. Once I went through that six-month process, I'd be back where I'd started, playing catch up—or was it dodge ball?—with my mortality. And flirting with Jackie O's fate—and maybe Nora's, Mary's, and Susan's. Was it time? It was time.

Me, My Hair, and I

In laboring to be beautiful, we worry not only about individual body parts—hair, eyes, lips, breasts—but the fear of "losing our looks" and the terror of looking our age. At exactly the time of the hair dye debacle, I had just finished editing an anthology of essays about women and their hair, *Me, My Hair and I: Twenty-seven Women Untangle an Obsession*, which would be published the following fall. In addition to editing the pieces and writing the introduction, I contributed an essay, "No, I Won't Go Gray," about my vanity and insistence on denying my age, which I paired next to Anne Kreamer's essay of giving up the dye precisely in order to feel her age.

By the day of the black dye debacle, it was too late to revise my essay, but that ill-fated chemical dunk was my last one. I began the long, awkward process of letting the salt in the salt and pepper take over while I refused to cut off the remaining dark ends because I was still ambivalent—oh, vanity!—about what I was doing.

While my paranoia about hair dye originated with an anecdote about Jackie Onassis and her lymphoma, the experience of editing *Me, My Hair and I* put me in touch with environmental journalist Ronnie Citron-Fink, who gave up hair dye when she learned about its dangers and investigated the matter in her book *True Roots: What Quitting Hair Dye Taught Me about Health and Beauty*. Between the huge NIH study and the revelations in this book—hair dye chemicals harm consumers, hairdressers, and the environment, into whose rivers these toxic fluids flow from the sinks of hair salons—my years of hypochondrial concern were not as far-fetched as some skeptical friends imagined.

It's Huge

In the waning days of June, I found an endocrinologist online who took my crap insurance and could see me right away in his office on Madison Avenue. He gasped when he felt the lump in my armpit—"It's huge!" he exclaimed, and I wonder to this day why he didn't order a biopsy of it right away instead of futzing around with my parathyroid. Still, he was serious and methodical, though puzzled by why I was such an emotional wreck. How could he have felt the huge lump and not been worried himself?

He had no idea why my upper chest burned, and he drew blood to test for a dreaded blood disease that I'd never heard of until he mentioned it. He also ordered a nuclear test of my neck for the following week, to see whether there was any evidence of a benign tumor on my parathyroid, which is what usually causes the elevated hormone levels I had had for twenty-plus years, and maybe accounted for some of my weird symptoms. I'd gotten the same nuclear test six years before, and there was no visible tumor. Because there was not an excess of calcium in my blood and hence no fatigue, the usual parathyroid surgery wasn't advised.

Ten days later, when the nuclear test came back with no evidence of a tumor—though my hormone level was three times higher than normal—the endocrinologist sent me to a top surgeon at Mount Si-nai. My appointment was for the following week, on July 15.

The day before that appointment, I returned to the radiology clin-ic and had a second sonogram of the lump. The same narrow room, a different technician and a different doctor, and James at the foot of the table with a notebook.

"I'm sure it's smaller," I bragged to the doctor, who was younger and taller than the previous one. He looked from the screen to the original report on a piece of paper.

"Uh, no," he said. "It's not."

"It *feels* smaller to me. When I touch it." Which I did every fifteen minutes.

"That's not what the scan shows."

"But how can . . ." How can that be, after more than a month of wheat grass, apple cider vinegar, and more jumps in the gym than a rabbit on the run?

"I'd recommend another follow-up in two to three weeks," the doc-tor said, and again I thought, *No one is alarmed, not the way they are if they see so much as a speck on the breast during a mammogram.* But I was going away in a few days for three weeks, so I figured I would get the next procedure—the biopsy or the PET scan—when I came back, in three-plus weeks.

"We'll send the report to your doctor in a few days," he said calmly as James and I left, buoyed by the absence of any expressed alarm. Life was sweet, I was fine—at least for the time being. The next day, a top surgeon would get to the bottom of my parathyroid problem. And a few days after that, we were getting out of Dodge, heading to a cottage on Martha's Vineyard we had rented eight months before.

It was a three-week working vacation where I was giving talks at two public libraries on college applications, meeting new clients, and seeing old friends. I had lived on the island for almost two years with my first husband at the end of our marriage, in the mid-1990s, and I had many layers of memories, some searingly painful, but it had been long enough for new layers to bury some of the old. That July, I was desperate to be away, to be far from the heat and stench of New York in summer and far from doctors who told me I was fine, who gasped when they felt the lump, and spoke in code that I did not yet know was code. It would be some time before I learned that when a radiologist says, Come back in two to three weeks, it's not good news; it's a two-alarm fire.

The Worm at the Core of Our Being

1. *Reality Frights.* A bear at the door. An icy road. A sick child. Rent you can't pay. Eviction. Divorce. A missing person.
2. *Distant But Scary.* A fear so remote it's a virtual impossibility. A meteor will strike my apartment building. The house will be swallowed by a sink hole.
3. *The Big One.* "The worm at the core of our being" was how philosopher William James put it—the knowledge we live with that we are going to die. Like a zoom lens on a camera that brings the subject closer or farther away, our awareness of that inescapable truth comes into focus and recedes. Day to ordinary day, the awareness is part of a wide shot, a view that encompasses the sky, the landscape, quotidian routines, fleeting fears. *Will I get to the store before it closes?* But real danger and serious illness draw the camera up close, so that fear takes up the entire screen.

What Brings You Here Today?

All I had was the address until we crossed 101st Street and saw the daunting silver letters on the façade of the modern glass and marble tower: Tisch Cancer Center. Why couldn't it just say "1470 Madison Avenue" or "Mount Sinai Hospital"? Even worse, two flights up, I had to check in beneath the words "Department of Surgical Oncology" stenciled on the wall. What was going on? Maybe the head and neck surgeon had an office here because they'd run out of room in the head and neck department? There had to be an explanation, I mean, other than, you know, *cancer*.

The doctor (tall, friendly, smiling, a beard and glasses, maybe fifty years old): "What brings you here today?" (Such good cheer; it was almost fun.)

The patient: "I have an elevated parathyroid but the nuclear test didn't show a tumor, and you're supposed to know what to do about that. Also, I've got this lump under my arm."

Doctor: "Well, let's have a look at the arm." (Arm outstretched, fingers probing my armpit, finding it in one swift grip.) "Let's get a biopsy on that. The doctor who does that procedure is here today." (More good cheer; bottoms up!)

Patient: "Now?!? Today?!?"

Doctor: "Yeah. His part is simple, just a fine needle aspiration that takes a few minutes. (Nodding amiably, turning to change gears and maybe make a phone call to contact the other doctor. Turning back to me.) "By the way, we'll deal with your parathyroid once we take care of this."

Patient (in mild panic, imagining vacation being canceled): "I'm going to Massachusetts in two days for three weeks. And what if . . . Can this wait for three weeks? I've got meetings scheduled and public appearances, and we've rented a house that's already paid for. But if it can't wait . . ."

Doctor: "That's fine. Not a problem. Let me explain what happens with the biopsy. If the first procedure finds any abnormal cells, that's all we know—abnormal cells—so we have to keep digging. I do a procedure called a core biopsy. I go a little deeper into the lymph node and extract more cells, though there usually aren't enough to do a diagnosis. We'll know whether we have enough in about a week. And if there aren't enough cells, we do an open biopsy—we remove a piece of the lymph node surgically. That's the only procedure that can give us a specific diagnosis."

Patient: "So even if I did the biopsy today, I wouldn't know the answer today, except if there are abnormal cells?"

Doctor: "That's right."

Patient: "The thing is, I don't want to find out I have cancer *today*. I mean, *today* because I'm going away, and I have all these appearances and appointments with clients. It's my livelihood. It's a working vacation."

I didn't want him to think I was a flibbertigibbet, someone who put her health on hold just to go to the beach.

Patient, again: "But I'm afraid it could be lymphoma."

Doctor: "Are you having night sweats?"

Patient: "No."

Doctor: "I don't think you have cancer. We can take care of this when you're back. Have a good vacation!"

Patient: "A working vacation."

And a three-week reprieve.

We made an appointment for biopsy number one, an FNA, for the next time we would all be back in the neighborhood: August 15. I left in high spirits. The doctor didn't think I had cancer—*how fucking great was that?*—and even if I proved him wrong, I wouldn't have to find out for a month. The cancer signs I passed on my way out of the building—the actual word affixed to the windows and walls—had just turned to dust.

Sleepless Nights

"Journey" in French is *la journée*, meaning a day's work, a day's travel—a definition now obsolete. Today, a journey is a trip from one place to another, usually involving some distance or significance. *A trip to the corner store versus a journey to our ancestral homeland.* Figuratively, a journey is "any process or progression likened to a journey, especially one that involves difficulties or personal development."

Speaking of journeys, I started Barnard College intending to be an art historian because I loved looking at art and studying the lives of artists, but after two or three courses, I understood that scholarship was not for me. When I was a sophomore, a professor responded to a personal essay I wrote about a Victorian novel and intuited that I wanted to write a novel of my own, which turned out to be a good idea I had never thought of. Soon writing was all I cared about, and as a college senior, I was lucky enough to have a tutorial with Elizabeth Hardwick. She was jolly and cynical and told me that the only thing she could really *do* for me was to suggest books I should read, and that I should read Rilke's *The Notebooks of Malte Laurids Brigge*, which I promptly did. Several times.

When I was at Barnard, Miss Hardwick, as I called her, was writing the novel that became *Sleepless Nights*. It was published in 1979, three years after I graduated. At a friend's apartment for dinner one night, she brandished her brand-new copy of the book, eager to read me a passage from the first few pages:

> Tickets, migrations, worry, property, debts, changes of name and changes back once more: these came about from reading many books. So from Kentucky to New York, to Boston, to Maine, to Europe, carried along on a river of paragraphs and chapters, of blank verse, of little books translated from the Polish and big books from the Russian—all consumed in a sedentary sleeplessness. Is that sufficient—never mind that it is the truth. It certainly hasn't the drama of: I saw the old, white-bearded frigate master on the dock and signed up for the journey. But after all, 'I' am a woman.

There was so much about the passage that was electrifying to us, though we focused on the shock of the white-bearded frigate master and the journey he signed up for, which plunged the paragraph into a distant century, into the history of literature, and then, in the last line, it swerved into the present feminist moment when we were working so hard to erase what was then the enormous gulf between men's and women's legal rights and opportunities. The narrator in Hardwick's book will not encounter the testosterone-driven drama of seafaring novels, but whose fault is that? Women have never been allowed on those docks, on those journeys, given access to those narratives. It was only earlier in that decade, 1974, that married women could have their own credit cards and lines of credit, and 1978 when it became illegal to fire a woman because she was pregnant. The Hardwick paragraph itself is a journey, starting with the abstract list and lurching every which way to the startling two final sentences.

My friend and I were at the start of our own life journeys, just a few years out of college, and both obsessed with words, sentences, and books like Hardwick's. We had no interest in medicine or law or money, nor at the time in getting married or having children. Most important, we were the grateful beneficiaries of the decade's older feminists; we were sixteen when the first issue of *Ms.* appeared in 1971. By the mid-1970s, I knew I wanted to be a novelist, though it would be many years before I wrote seriously and began to publish. And many more years before I wanted children. My work was always more important.

It surprises me how often I've remembered those moments in my friend's living room with *Sleepless Nights* and especially the shared frisson of those few lines from the novel, the unexpected comparison of men's journeys to women's. This would lead, decades later, to an interest in accounts of so many journeys, among them Bashō's work of travel and haiku, *Narrow Road to the Deep North*, published in Japan in 1702. My interest in Bashō grew when the novelist Howard Norman did his own reprise of Bashō's journey in 2007 and wrote about it for *National Geographic*.

As I read Howard's account now, I'm entranced by the depth of his fascination with Bashō, by the details and digressions that tell Bashō's story and his own parallel journey, and by the chutzpah of Howard's two-month trek. Had he been afraid of anything that would have frightened me on that trip? Illness, falls, animal bites, taxi accidents— I had quite a list of potential calamities. But I wanted to see what he saw, to be a person whose curiosity eclipses her fear.

Had it been easy for Howard Norman to show up on the dock with the white-bearded frigate master and set off on his adventure? And was my own fear sex-linked—a woman alone far from home? Why wasn't my husband part of this fantasy, this imagined adventure? I pondered these questions as I discovered a ten-day tour of Bashō's trek, thinking, *Maybe, maybe one day.* As romantic as Howard's expedition was, as much as I wish I had the *kishkes* to do what he did, I would never sign up for the extended journey he took. I don't need the hero's journey.

But I wonder: Is the opposite of the hero's journey the victim's journey?

And was that the journey I was on now?

The Word "Mismeasured"

A message appeared in my patient portal as I was packing to leave New York for Martha's Vineyard: the sonogram report from the radiology lab with the briefest of notes from Sylvie, the nurse practitioner: "Here are the test results."

The report heading minced no words: "Right axilla palpable abnormality."

But it was another word, far down in the report, that was an even bigger surprise. The text explained that this sonogram and the previous one had been done on different machines, but even with that factor, the initial lymph nodes, studied on June 13, had been mismeasured. *Mismeasured*? They were *larger* than originally stated. And in the time from when they were mismeasured on June 13 to July 14, the larger one had grown from 3.3 x 1.6 x 2.0 cm to 3.7 x 1.6 x 2.6 cm.

I shook as I read and remembered the words of the radiologist mom that had been so reassuring a month before. "There's nothing to worry about unless it's three centimeters or bigger," she'd said, and we both sighed with relief when I read that my own were so much smaller. But we had sighed in error, though the error wasn't our own. The bigger one had always been bigger than three centimeters, but no one had known it, which meant that my problem had never been my anxiety, which meant that the lump had always been a "palpable abnormality." Yet two days before, the surgeon had said, "I don't think you have cancer." Had I made a terrible mistake, not getting the biopsy two days ago? Yet it would only have been the results from the FNA that day—nothing definitive. But who was I kidding?

Only myself, for as long as possible.

And there was this calculation, this observation I kept repeating to myself: *None of these doctors was panicking, none of them insisting that I stay in the city and cancel my trip. If they weren't panicking, why should I?*

Country Life

Off we went to the cottage on Lambert's Cove Road, a thousand feet from the beach in one direction and, in the other direction, the pond where I like to swim. James spent most days sitting on the porch reading, his books spread out on the glass-topped table, the little house surrounded by towering trees and cloudless deep blue skies. I got up early most days and went bike riding alone on the other side of the island, pedaling down Ocean Drive before the beach crowds showed up, and on back roads that ran along Katama Bay. I nodded to the occasional runner, to dog walkers and stroller pushers, and marveled that the air was soft against my skin and that I was far enough from the city to shed some of my urban survivalist armor. I still didn't know exactly what was wrong with me, but the top layers of my anxiety had burned off like fog in sunlight. The worm at the core of my being had slithered away for the time being.

We are such creatures of the city, James and I, it always surprises me that we collapse into this life so naturally. The narrow, winding roads, the outdoor shower, the incredible stillness. We saw old friends and did not mention what was going on. We did sweet country things: walked down our winding two-lane road to splash in the sound, bought vegetables and eggs at the honor-system farm stand, ate strawberry rhubarb pie that had won first prize at the Agricultural County Fair, grilled fish and yellow squash out back, and ate dinner on the porch, blissed out by the tastes of the food and the trees we had to stretch our necks to see. Our urban selves would return in a flash as we drove off to movies, concerts, and lectures by people who live a few subway stops from us in New York. So much for the privations of our simple country life.

The only medical professional I spoke to was our friend Kate, a retired nurse practitioner and one of the wise medical people I know. During a visit to the remote house in the woods that she shares with her writer husband, I told her my story and tried to convince her that there was still some chance this was not what I feared it was. And she kindly played along. I mentioned the bad news but stressed the good. "The surgeon said he didn't think I had cancer" and "No one is insisting I drop everything and report to Memorial Sloan Kettering."

"That is good news, Liz!"

"You don't *not* get news like that every day, do you?"

"You sure don't."

We laughed and laughed, but I did not let her touch the palpable abnormality in my right axilla—because I knew she would have an opinion about it, and I didn't want to put her in the position of knowing something about me that I didn't want to know myself or of making her feel that she had to lie. Or that she had to tell me the truth. I was sure that the surgeon in New York had lied to me, but would I have preferred that he had said, "You probably do have cancer, but we can wait till you come back to treat it"?

Drop a pin in this question.

"I Don't Think You Have Cancer"

On our way home, we stopped in Boston, where I still had a gynecologist to see for my annual checkup. After she examined me and heard what was going on, she said, "I don't think you have cancer."

What did these doctors *see* when they said this to me? My complexion? My energy? My fondest wish? Or was it just a dumb throwaway, a feel-better statement that cost them nothing?

A few months later, I would complain about these "I don't think you have cancer" comments to a psychiatrist, who was prescribing me anti-depressants because I did, after all—of course I did!—have cancer. I had expected to hear this kind of throwaway assurance from friends, but not from doctors. The shrink's cheery yet matter-of-fact response startled me: "Liz, you know that doctors have a hard time giving people bad news."

Yeah, I'd read about that. And now I'd seen it for myself. Good to know, and directly from someone in the club, that I hadn't been hallucinating. I was too depressed—and too committed to conserving my energy—to point out the sad commentary in his remark. Not to mention that I was mildly offended that he'd taken the doctors' side in gaslighting me for what turned out to be months. By the time the shrink and I had this conversation in his office in the Department of Psychiatry at Mount Sinai, I knew the truth, and I was not at all sure how the rest of this drama—that is to say, my life—was going to play out. I was in no position to be indignant, and I did not have the energy for it either. Plus, I was there for the drugs, not the conversation.

For months afterwards, I was puzzled that so many doctors had tiptoed so daintily around the possibility of cancer, which brings with it the dark clouds of mortality. But it would be much longer before I understood that their reluctance was a feature of their training and outlook, not a bug. Many of them were as eager to delay mentioning the word as I was eager to delay hearing it.

Part *Two*

"What the Doctor Said"

August 15, 2017. Biopsy number one. I'm sent to a doctor's office in an apartment building a few blocks from Mount Sinai. The pathologist, a roving pathologist, comes on Tuesdays and rents this space. No receptionist, no patients, no lights on—everyone must've been on vacation, the only light a bit of sun through the grimy first-floor windows and the ancient metal Venetian blinds.

"Are you sure this is the right place?" James said.

"We'll find out soon enough."

A young woman appeared in the waiting area and took me, alone, into a distant exam room where I met a compact Asian man in shirtsleeves—no suit jacket, no white medical coat. Right away, I noticed a microscope on the counter, not a common sight. Otherwise, an ordinary exam room with a few syringes laid out on a plastic tray and a portable sonogram machine. The woman handed him objects as he situated me on the table and asked me to raise my right arm over my head. He pressed the infamous spot with a wand and looked at the nearby screen.

"There are three enlarged lymph nodes," he said quietly.

Oh, Christ, I was a goner. The third one in the last month.

"I'm going to insert a needle into the one closest to the surface and extract some cells and look at them under the microscope. If there's nothing problematic, I'll go into the lymph node under it. And if there's nothing, I'll go to the third. Ready?"

The pinching under my arm did not last as long as I thought it would. With my eyes closed, because I couldn't bear to catch a glimpse of his expression when he looked under the microscope, I could sense the doctor step away from the table and could hear faint sounds that must have been the slide going into the microscope, the adjustments, the assessment.

"Another?" the assistant asked. She meant another slide, another poke farther down into my lymph nodes.

The next sound I heard was him saying, "Uh uh." I knew he had seen all he needed to see in the first aspiration.

"Why don't you sit up?"

I swung my legs over the side of the table. What would he say? How would he say it? This would always be the before-and-after moment, and I wanted to remember it.

"When there are three swollen lymph nodes," he began, "it's a sign of lymphoma. And I'm seeing abnormal cells on the slide."

"I want to get my husband." I slid off the table and walked a few steps to the door, calling "James" into the long, dark hallway. Nothing the doctor said surprised me, but I didn't want to hear it alone. As James came into view, I met his eye, shook my head and wrinkled up my nose—to prepare him.

"It looks like lymphoma," the doctor said to us, "but I can't tell from this slide what kind. There are dozens of variations." I had read that there are sixty—or was it eighty? "I'll send the results across the street to the doctor. You have an appointment with him now, is that right?"

I nodded.

"He'll do a deeper biopsy that will determine what it is precisely."

I said, "Thank you" to the doctor, and as soon as I did, lines from the Raymond Carver poem, "What the Doctor Said," splashed into my memory like a stone into water—about the strangeness of saying "thank you" to the doctor who'd just told him his lung cancer is "bad in fact real bad." I had read the poem aloud at my father's memorial service—my father who had died of lung cancer at seventy-five after a lifetime of smoking. I had always believed that I would outlive him because I took good care of myself, down to my organic dental floss.

What the Other Doctor Said

We were kind of numb and kind of relieved and indisputably terrified. All I remember about walking up Madison Avenue to 101st Street, back to the Tisch Cancer Center, is that we did not speak because this was the news we had expected to hear. Is there an emotion unique to the situation, a situation so common that there should be? The way you feel when you learn after months of worry that you have what might be a fatal illness but you're not sure yet how fatal it is? All I remember from that brief journey is that as we went up in the crowded elevator to Surgical Oncology, I said to James, "I'm going to tell him he was wrong." It would be an icebreaker when we got to the surgeon's office. And I felt that it was all I had left in the way of personal power now that this disease had officially been thrust on me—my puny accusation, a wee bit of wit. He had all of medicine on his side.

"Wrong about what?" the surgeon said brightly when I leveled my charge, in what I thought was a vaguely jokey voice. "Well, doc, looks like you were wrong," but I skipped the "doc." He was a good-natured man with an all-American, white-bread name and a somewhat alien Midwestern friendliness.

"You said you didn't think I had cancer," I said to him, "but I do."

"The pathologist found some abnormal cells. That doesn't mean it's cancer."

What? This couldn't be happening, could it? More games about my condition, more unwillingness to tell me what was going on when ten minutes ago I had said "thank you" to the man who'd told me it looked like lymphoma?

"I've seen all kinds of things. We won't know for sure until we get the results from either the core or the open biopsy. Let's do the core biopsy now. I'll tell my assistant to get ready."

I never imagined I would have such a complicated relationship with a doctor who wasn't a therapist. Instead of us now traveling on the same train, the train of reality, his latest comments had the feel of a weird comedy routine, or was it *The Twilight Zone*? James and I swapped faces of disbelief, speechless at the doctor's noncommittal message, after preparing all summer for the news we had just heard. Hadn't we reached a new level of candor that finally matched the science of the situation? Did the doctor really think I needed to be cancer-coddled at this point?

He returned suited up in a baby blue full-body apron and plastic, AIDS-proof goggles, and carrying a small tray of assorted hypodermic needles, including one big enough for an elephant, with a tiny hook at the point of the needle. I turned my head away, shut my eyes, and decided to skip my questions.

"I'm going to inject you with Lidocaine to reduce some of the discomfort," he said. "It'll take a few minutes for the numbness to take effect." One quick jab into my armpit, and he disappeared again, and I braced for the next jab, which I knew would not be as inconsequential. James asked me how I was doing, and I closed my eyes and shook my head as my sister's Buddhist chant floated up into the distraction warehouse in my brain. *Nam Myoho Renge Kyo*. Or whatever it was. I mouthed the words or mis-mouthed them over and over until I heard the doctor return, and I braced for the elephant needle with a tiny hook at the end.

"This shouldn't hurt too much. I'm just going to—"

"Don't tell me about it, OK, just do it." *Nam Myoho Renge Kyo. Nam Myoho Renge Kyo. Nam Myoho Renge Kyo. Nam Myoho Renge Kyo.* I was getting the hang of it, even if I had no idea what it meant.

"Done," the doctor said. "Not too bad, was it?"

What I Wanted to Say to the Doctor

He unsuited and took a small leather date book from his breast pocket and flipped through it. "These results should be back in two or three days—by Friday. I'll be going on vacation Friday, so I'll have someone call you with the results." A few more pages. "I'll be back the day after Labor Day—September fifth." September fifth? Today was August fifteenth. "We can meet then to discuss the results. In case we don't get enough cells to make a determination, which is usually what happens, we should schedule an open biopsy for . . . let's see. The first day I can schedule the operating room is . . . Looks like September eleventh. We should have the results from that by September nineteenth. That will be the definitive diagnosis. Got all those dates?"

He had just moved the goalposts to the other end of the field, and I was speechless, but what could I say—how dare you go on vacation? "I have to wait another month to find out what this is?"

"We might know something Friday, but it's unlikely."

"But what if this is cancer? Don't I need to be treated?"

"Yes, if it *is*."

"I mean now. I mean soon. Now there are three swollen lymph nodes."

September nineteenth would be more than three months since I first felt the lump. What if this was spreading to my spleen, to my bone marrow? I had read that lower back pain was a symptom, and itching too, because whatever is coursing through your blood makes your skin itch. That morning I'd felt a pain in my right shoulder—the *bones* of my shoulder. That could mean it was in my bone marrow. And where exactly *was* my spleen? And what if I had cancer some-where else and the lymph node was a metastasis? What if whatever this was had leapt from stage one in June to stage three or four in September? And he was going on vacation?

This is what happened thirty-eight years ago to Deena—such a long delay diagnosing her breast cancer that it spread to her lymph nodes and she had to have twenty-eight of them removed. She had tried to sue the doctor but she couldn't get hold of the X-rays. When she'd told me these stories years before, I vowed I would never let that happen to me. And here I was.

"If it is cancer, the tumors grow very slowly," the doctor said. "They can grow over five years. There's plenty of time."

My radiology report said they had grown in a month and now there was a third, but what choice did I have except to go along with this schedule? I couldn't very well find another doctor at the end of August. Yet I had to advocate for myself. I couldn't be one of those patients who just nods.

"What did you mean," I ventured, "when you said that this might not be cancer when the other doctor said it was lymphoma?"

"He said it *suggested* lymphoma, but fine needle biopsies don't pro-vide specific diagnoses. We don't know the results until we have the report from the pathologist. In twenty years, I've seen all kinds of things happen, things that surprised me."

Like what? I wanted to say. Like cancer that wasn't cancer after all? Really? How often does that happen? But he was edging his way out of the room, and I didn't want to be a pest. Our time was up. Today was Tuesday, and Friday he was leaving for vacation. In another month, there could be four swollen nodes. Are they still called swollen if they are swollen with malignant cells? Are they called tumors then or have they always been tumors?

"Someone will call me Friday with the results?"

"Yes," he said, sidling closer to the door.

"And if there's something that needs to be taken care of in the results, is there someone here while you're gone?"

"Yes, one of my colleagues is covering for me."

Out he went as I slid off the examining table, the paper crackling beneath me, and into James' arms. We were in a state beyond words, beyond sad, scared, and furious.

A Missing Can of Beans

No one called me from the doctor's office on Friday when the results of the core biopsy came in. For all of my New York moxie, I was too afraid to call the doctor's office on Monday, Tuesday, or any other day to have another dishonest encounter with another medical professional whose tone of voice I would try to read for clues as to the information that biopsy number two had revealed, and that the person wouldn't want to tell me. Instead, I just waited. As I had waited all summer. Seventeen more days from the day the call didn't come. I was sure the results of the test were ghastly—a definitive diagnosis that no one covering for the doctor had the gumption to tell me.

I was like a kid waiting for the school year to end or for my birthday to come, wondering how I would trick the time into passing more quickly.

I kept busy. I worked on Skype with clients applying to college, walked up and down Broadway buying groceries, rode my bike in Riverside Park, called friends, and called my sister. I cried. I wondered what I would say to my clients and their parents if I had to stop working, so I set up extra meetings before school started so that we'd finish what they were working on sooner rather than later. Another line of worry was what to say to new people who called and wanted to hire me. "I might have cancer" was not what any of them wanted to hear. Another line of worry was money. If I couldn't get more clients and my medical bills went sky high, what would I do? I composed emails to friends in my head, asking if they would consider contributing to a fund. I didn't need money yet, but who knew where this might lead?

I called friends who had had cancer and asked what they had been through, and their stories and their recoveries soothed my frazzled nerves. I called my friend S., whose partner's family was practically a cancer cluster and who was himself something of a cancer hotline. He told me about a woman he knew who went for a routine physical, at the end of which she was ordered to Memorial Sloan Kettering that day and could not even go home for a toothbrush. There she stayed for a month, and we agreed that whatever the bleep was wrong with me, that wasn't the kind of cancer I had. S. also said that this woman's shit of a husband abandoned her during her illness.

"Liz, instead of worrying about cancer," he said, "maybe you should worry that your husband will leave you," which he could say because we had been friends for thirty years, and I appreciated his joke almost as much as I appreciated my husband's devotion. I also really liked hearing that the woman who'd been ordered to MSK without a toothbrush was fine now.

The seventeen days did eventually pass, and we showed up as scheduled in Surgical Oncology on September 5, bracing for The Awful Truth. I was ready to take it between the eyes. The doctor pushed open the door with a smile on his face and said brightly, "Hi, how are you today?"

"What were the results of the biopsy?"

"There weren't any. Not enough cells to tell us anything."

"No one called me."

"Sorry about that." His voice as light as could be, as though the unmade phone call had been about a missing can of beans. "Looks like we're on schedule for the open biopsy next week. Let's see. Yes, September 11. My assistant will give you the information about checking into the hospital and what you need to do" and blah blah blah blah blah.

To him, this was routine, another patient, another appointment in Surgical Onc, another phone call someone forgot to make. This was what he did all day long, the way I move words around a page, and maybe if I were a champion chanter instead of a part-time, drive-by chanter, I'd have had a response that was enlightened, mellow, full of grace. But I was enraged, and I knew that expressing even an ounce of my indignation would be a profound waste of time. It would remind me that the source of whatever personal power I have—the power to express myself, to use words effectively—was of no value whatsoever in the face of cancer or whatever was wrong with me, even if this doctor refused to give it a name. I knew that if I expressed half the fury I felt, I would end up feeling humiliated and, if it was possible, more powerless than I already felt.

Which is why I said nothing as I seethed.

On Being Ill

In her long essay *On Being Ill*, Virginia Woolf thought it strange "that illness has not taken its place with love and battle and jealousy among the prime themes of literature" when we consider "how common illness is, how tremendous the spiritual change that it brings, how astonishing, when the lights of health go down, the undiscovered countries that are then disclosed."

When she wrote this in 1930, illness had not been entirely absent from stories (*The Yellow Wallpaper, The Death of Ivan Ilyich, Death in Venice, The Magic Mountain,* Chekhov stories, William Carlos Williams' *Doctor Stories*), but in the nearly one hundred years since, it has moved from the sidelines to somewhere near the center of many writers' gazes. For one thing, we live long enough to tell the stories of our maladies and our recovery. For another, there's so much more to say. So much more even since 1978, when Sontag published *Illness as Metaphor*, in which she compared figures of speech used to describe tuberculosis before it was cured to cancer as it was described in the 1970s. She does a brilliant job tracing the history of metaphorizing illnesses and arguing that as long as a deathly illness is not curable, people will reach for metaphors to explain its power. TB's early metaphors romanticized the affliction and the sufferers. Said Thoreau, who had TB: "Death and disease are often beautiful, like . . . the hectic glow of consumption." By contrast, cancer's metaphors invoked war, battle, and the certainty of defeat. It's described, Sontag writes, as "an evil, invincible predator, not just a disease." The thrust of her argument is that the negative, defeatist language turns patients away from seeking treatment, and that if the language were renounced or just put aside, *ignored*, the fear of treatment, of *going into battle*, would diminish.

It's a persuasive argument as arguments go—stop comparing illnesses to other things, and you can go about getting treatment without feeling that you are *waging a war*. But as a practical matter, how do we just give up making comparisons? It might be as difficult as giving up smoking cigarettes, which we know we need to do too, but which, if you are inclined that way—if you are smoker, if you are a human who makes comparisons—is immensely difficult to do. I use the smoking metaphor to argue against her use of metaphor—because that's how natural it is to reach for metaphors.

She argues: When we make illness a metaphor, and that metaphor involves war, we too easily let it dominate our plans. But could it be that the metaphors merely matched the enemy they described? That in the 1970s, patients and the disease were unquestionably at war, and that in those years, cancer was likely to win, regardless of the colorful comparisons you made or refrained from making?

Was it the metaphors that kept—and keep—people from seeking treatment or was it the disease itself, the disruptions to our lives, the requirement that we confront our mortality, undergo ghastly treatments, and face uncertain outcomes? Doesn't cancer have to lose some of its actual power to kill before we can strip it of metaphors or find metaphors that are less intimidating?

Speaking of metaphors, Grace Paley asked, "Who is the boss of beauty?"

Today I wonder: Who is the boss of cancer metaphors? Have cancer metaphors changed since 1978, now that a few battles have been won and a few defeats have been delayed, not just for weeks or months but years and sometimes decades?

Oh, for the time when cancer is, say, a walk in the park.

Which One Do You Have?

So many miraculous advances in science and medicine since 1930, but we are still very much at war with cancer, despite decisive victories on the front lines. Or should I write that sentence to emphasize what's improved rather than what has not? There *are* real triumphs though they may not be broad or deep enough yet to lay waste to centuries of warlike metaphors. How to measure metaphors anyway? One way is in Siddhartha Mukherjee's monumental history of cancer, *The Emperor of All Maladies*, published in 2010. He uses the word "battle" forty-four times, and "war" about a hundred times, mostly metaphorically.

Still, declines in death rates from cancer have been dramatic during the last three decades. Overall, deaths from cancer dropped twenty-seven percent from 1991 to 2017—though the figure is largely attributable to declines in smoking cigarettes and hence in lung cancer. Advances in breast cancer detection and new treatments have meant dramatic declines in death rates since 1989, though the successes are not shared across racial lines: Black women under fifty are twice as likely to die from breast cancer as white women.

Yet Hodgkin's disease, the type of lymphoma that I believed extinguished Sue Briskman in 1972—though I learned in 2022 that it was non-Hodgkin's—is now curable. Not just manageable but curable—

the *ne plus ultra* of cancers. If you are going to get it, I learned on Google, Hodgkin's is the one to get, the brass ring you want to snatch as you sail by on the merry-go-round of life interrupted. Unfortunately, though, it was not the one I got.

"As I understand it," said a woman I am not often in touch with, "there are two kinds of lymphoma." She meant Hodgkin's and non, though there are about eighty varieties under those umbrellas. "And one is much worse than the other. Which one do you have?"

"I have the one that's much worse," I said, hoping she would hear the indelicacy in her question and, if not that, the edge in my answer, though I have no reason to think she heard either.

All this time later, her question still irks me. Yet I don't want to be in the habit of collecting grievances because not everyone knows what it's like to dwell in the house of cancer. And if they do, their dwelling place is different from mine. The vast variety of cancers and the proximity to so much suffering and uncertainty when I was barely managing my own, were some of the reasons I never considered a cancer support group. On the other hand, I was lucky enough to have Deena in my Friend Corner.

"It will make you humble," she told me once I had the diagnosis. Deena, a nearly forty-year breast cancer survivor, was my cancer role model, my cancer guru. "And you will learn something from it," she added.

I vowed to be on the *qui vive*.

"It Could Have Been Worse"

In the surgeon's exam room on September 19, 2017, I was obsessed with imagining his face as he walked through the door to give me—at long last—the definitive results more than three months after I discovered the lumps. We barely knew each other, the doctor and I, but we had a complicated relationship by then, built on alternating layers of trust and deception, thrust and parry, as least as I saw it. He, I imagine, did not think much about the nature of what passed between us, unless it involved the specifics of my healthcare. At least I hope he didn't. When he left my exam room, his next appointment was with another patient, another set of problems to solve. Patients left behind had only our terror for company.

I was forthright with him about my fears, but his candor was much more measured, like a parent doling out trinkets of information about the facts of a life to a small child. On the one hand I was complicit because I didn't ask a million Deena-style questions. But when I did, his refrain was that he simply didn't know what the lump was and couldn't say until the biopsy results were in.

When he had operated on me the week before, intending to remove a chunk of lymph node to be biopsied, he explained right afterwards that he took out the entire lymph node. Another doctor on the team walked past and said, "It was three-quarters as big as a golf ball!" with a lilt of delighted wonder in her voice. She smiled. The surgeon smiled. He was sitting with me in the recovery room, pretending to hang out. I was surprised to see him there since it's usually nurses in these places.

I was still a high on the Valium drip, happy to be alive, and happy to be eating graham crackers because I hadn't eaten anything for almost twenty-four hours. "I called James," the doctor said cheerily. "He'll be here soon. I asked how his class on Wagner was." He was still smiling, and I knew this was a dead giveaway, accent on *dead*. I remembered hearing that Sue Briskman's parents had bought her something extravagant once she was sick, and she figured it meant she was going to die.

Should I ask why he took out the whole lymph node when that wasn't the plan? Hadn't he told me sometimes people's arms swell up when lymph nodes are removed? Wasn't there a name for that—and would that happen to me now? What did the node he removed look like? Did cancerous nodes look different from others? Couldn't a doctor tell just by looking that there was something wrong with mine? True to form, I asked nothing. And true to form, he answered only the questions he was asked, like that parent whose kid wants to know where babies come from. *Tell them only what you think they need to know.* We both did a masterful job ignoring the elephant in the middle of the recovery room. C-A-N-C-E-R.

I ate graham crackers and chatted amiably, and the doctor pretended to be interested. The longer he sat there, the worse I knew it was. The lymph node must have had a skull and crossbones on it.

When James appeared, the doctor smiled and chatted some more, as though he'd just removed a cute baby instead of a tumor. He might as well have bought me a pony. Or a yacht. Perhaps like poor Sue I had only months to live.

A week later in his office, when the pathology report would be finished, I wanted to be ready. I wanted to be able to read the surgeon's face before he said a thing. If he asked me how I was instead of just spitting out the results, I would gape at him in rage. The exam room where we waited was small, and I sat at the edge of the paper-covered exam table facing the door. James and I were silent, bracing ourselves for a blow—or a confirmation of the blows we had already received. The space from my knees to the door was no more than six feet.

Why did the expression on the doctor's face matter so much when he opened the door? Why did I think of nothing but that as I sat and waited for fifteen then twenty then twenty-five minutes past the time of our appointment? Was it because I felt he had toyed with me for so long, kept up a cheery patter instead of admitting that cancer was a possibility and this, finally, was the moment of truth? Would he enter the room with a smile on his face and then tell me I had cancer? Or would his expression match the truth of what he was most likely to say?

A gentle knock and then he was there, with a man much younger behind him, a medical student or a resident. The doctor was tall and slightly hunched over and wore a pinstriped suit and a starched white shirt. He was not smiling, and we were looking directly at each other. "It is lymphoma," he said softly.

"Hodgkin's?" I didn't know then that only young people got that.

"Non-Hodgkin's." He looked quickly over the piece of paper in his hands. "It could have been worse—it's not a metastasis from another cancer. Here's the pathology report and the name of the doctor who's head of our lymphoma treatment. You should call him right away."

The words "right away" did not get lost in the shuffling of our dazed selves walking out of the exam room and staggering down the antiseptic hallway to the elevator. Perhaps I exaggerate "staggering." We walked. We did not come close to falling. We were victorious only in that we finally knew what the hell was wrong with me, though there would be much more to find out, much more to make us stumble, lose our breath, and want to sleep with the lights on.

For the doctor, it was all in a day's work: the results of the biopsy. Here's what you do next. Call the guy who is next in line to treat you *right away*.

It had been three months and ten days since I first consulted a doctor about the lump in my arm.

Verklempt

We emerged from the Tisch Cancer Center into a humid, overcast September day, sidewalks bustling with people going into and coming out of so many medical towers, being pushed in wheelchairs, gripping walkers, hanging onto the arms of sturdier relatives, many of them as *verklempt* as we were. The news was not shocking, but I believe we were in shock, if only because we had to adjust to the state of *knowing* rather than blundering through each day for months in a cloud of fear. The loved one on her deathbed vs. the loved one dead. A different reality, though not unexpected.

On the corner of 96th and Madison: "You sure you'll be able to teach?" I asked James, due downtown in half an hour to lead a class on Wagner's *Ring Cycle*. Not exactly a breezy counterpoint to the opera of illness and gloom in which we had starring roles.

"I'll be fine," he said. The hint of a smile. "I think." The light gone out of his eyes, but I knew his preternatural powers of concentration and compartmentalization, and his love of teaching, would carry him through.

James went east to the subway station on Lexington, and I walked west to the crosstown bus. I had too much nervous energy to sit in a cab, and I suppose I wanted to pretend that this was a day like any other. I wanted to pretend that even knowing the hard truth, I could board the bus, one foot in front of the other, with only a new to-do list and my sister's voice on the phone and then her silence.

Another Thing about Illness

There is a rule of fiction writing—which means that no one is there to enforce it and it is easily broken—that two stories should always be going on at once. Maybe it's a plot and a subplot or only a conflict and a secondary conflict. Maybe it's the layers of well-mannered strife playing out in *Pride and Prejudice* or blocks of chaos erupting in Melville's *Moby Dick*. The thing about serious illness in real life is that it easily becomes the only plot, next to which other stories are background noise, trivia, junk mail, another call from another computer saying that your car warranty has expired even though you don't own a car. The thing about serious illness is that we all become Ahab chasing the white whale—with apologies to Susan Sontag for daring to compare.

"Give Me Your Phone Number, Honey"

Number one on my to-do list: email pathology report to friend who used to run Memorial Sloan Kettering and ask him for referral. Number two: phone Mount Sinai doc who runs lymphoma treatment department.

"His next appointment," said the woman who answered, "is in two months."

It was almost funny, like a punchline to a long, cruel joke. Or maybe I mean it was Kafkaesque, a word I plucked from mothballs for the occasion. For a long moment I was tongue-tied. "Two months?" Maybe I hadn't heard right.

"Yes."

"But I've been a patient at the hospital since—" I started and thought better of it. "I think there's a better offer for me somewhere in the universe." The line unspooled without my knowing exactly where it would end up.

I dropped the phone on the couch and looked for the scrap of paper on which I'd written the name of a doctor who had treated a friend's mother.

"I'm sure he's retired," my friend had recently warned, "because he was old when he treated her fifteen years ago. She was seventy-two when she was diagnosed, and died at eighty-five of something else. He was *the best*."

Seventy-seven but not out of the game. His bio and Google reviews described a legend. Within minutes, I was on the phone with his receptionist. "Give me your phone number, honey." Her voice—kindly, frail, not what I expected at a medical superstar's office. "The doctor likes to talk to new patients himself. He'll call you later today." The doctor's attentiveness more startling than the diagnosis itself.

An hour later, another happy turn in the story. My former-head-of-MSK friend wrote to say, "As I'm sure they told you at Mount Sinai, this is a common form of lymphoma with several treatments." This was much more concrete than "It could have been worse," and I repeated it in the group email I was writing to friends and family. "I could help you get an appointment," he went on, "with lymphoma specialists at Weill Cornell or Memorial Sloan Kettering, both of which have excellent records with this condition. You can also just make an appointment yourself; both are always seeking new patients."

It was a seesaw of a day, bouncing between emotional extremes at a brisk pace, intermixed with emails sent and received. And this incredible news from my friend—that what I had was treatable! Why didn't that end the drama—the encounter with my mortality—right there? It certainly lowered the temperature, but I knew there was more to this process than the first diagnosis. I knew I had to be "staged," and I was certain the cancer had spread because it had taken so long to diagnose. Good news, bad news, uncertain news.

A few minutes after James got back from teaching, we had to prepare for an encounter we had hoped to avoid until we got more used to the news ourselves.

Violin Strapped to Her Back

Emily texted us to ask if she could stay the following night. She had a rehearsal the morning after in the city. The last we'd told her, in July, the swollen thing in my armpit was nothing to worry about. We hadn't wanted to burden her with all of our uncertainty.

"Yes, fine to stay tomorrow," James texted back, "but can you Facetime with us soon?"

There is a lot James and I don't say to each other because we agree about so much that it would be redundant. There was no need to say how much we dreaded having to tell Emily. It's hard enough to drop the news on friends and other relatives, but, I was learning, a special anguish comes with telling children, even adult children. I was the first of her three parents to come home with a cancer diagnosis—the youngest of the three by eight years, and the one who, in my idle projections, was statistically meant to outlast the other two. But as we waited those fifteen minutes until Emily said we could call her, I don't know if we were both thinking about Janet, James' sister who had died eight years before of lung cancer, after hanging on miraculously for six years from the time she got a stage four diagnosis. Would I be the next woman in the family to die too young?

"We got some news today," James began, when we saw her on the computer screen.

"About the swollen lymph node in my arm," I chimed in. "We didn't tell you everything as it was going on because we didn't know the outcome, and we didn't want you to worry. But we just got the diagnosis."

She is a reserved soul and a performer, someone who can shut off what she needs to shut off and play a complicated instrument for many hours a day. I didn't think she would break down in front of us when she heard, and she didn't—she was quiet, she listened—but I wanted her to know before she arrived the next day, wanted her to share the news with her partner, Scott, before she arrived. I imagined she would be nervous coming into the apartment, a kind of stage fright, until she got through the door, the way you have to brace yourself to enter the hospital room of someone who is very sick.

"I don't want you to be afraid to see me. I mean, it's okay if you are, but I hope you're not. The doctors say it's very treatable, and I'm waiting for a call back from one of the leading doctors in the world. I'm going to be okay." I believed what I was saying as long as I was talking to her, but I knew it might be otherwise.

I could see Emily was holding back, pursing her lips. It was Facetime, and the image wasn't crystal clear. Were tears forming in her eyes? Was Scott there for her to go to when she got off the computer?

"We wanted to tell you before you came, so you wouldn't be surprised."

She didn't say much—a lot to absorb—but I remember her arrival the next afternoon, coming in the door with her violin strapped to her back, pulling her rolling suitcase, hugging me still in her coat, the instrument still wrapped around her shoulders. I could feel she was crying. "I'm going to be okay," I said, "and I have the best doctor in the world. I'll tell you about my phone call with him." I had plenty of people to pour my heart and my fears out to—I preferred to comfort her. And the story of my phone call with the doctor had been dazzling.

Cancer Is the New Puberty

He had phoned at six-twenty the night before—just hours after I cold-called him. His baritone voice matched his stature but everything else was a surprise, especially the warmth in his voice that sounded like he was just starting out as a doctor, not coming up on fifty years in business. He wanted me to read him a few lines of numbers from the pathology report. Every third or fourth number, he'd say, "That's good," and when I was through, he said, "I think this is curable."

He gave me a list of tests I needed, including a PET scan and instructions on how to order another set of slides for his pathologists—essential to determine the treatment. We made an appointment for October 4—two weeks later. His office was on East 70th Street, half a block from Weill Cornell.

Then it was time to kibitz. "You're a writer. Have you ever thought about writing a book about people who are left-handed?"

"Well, no, actually."

"What about people with red hair? That could be very interesting."

"Maybe. Maybe so. Hadn't considered that either."

"Just some ideas. Now, don't worry, dear. I think you're going to be fine. I'll call you tomorrow."

I was speechless all over again—at my good fortune, after months of zombie medicine. A doctor who believed whatever I had was "curable," or at least that was what he said to me over the phone. I understood he needed a lot more information about the state of my body before our meeting. And I understood—more than ever—that doctors say all kinds of things that aren't exactly true. But I didn't go into those hard-earned lessons when I recounted this phone call to Emily.

I did what Cole Porter's song tells us to do: ac-cent-tchu-ate the posi-tive.

Nor did I tell her about the rest of that first night after getting the diagnosis, that right before we went to sleep, I got an email from a friend who had dwelled in the house of cancer himself a few years before. "Overheard recently," he wrote: "Cancer is the new puberty." James and I laughed out loud.

Could it be time for a new cancer metaphor? The message here was the opposite of the war and battle metaphors that Sontag had blasted in 1978: *everyone goes through it and survives.* We knew it wasn't true—cancer deaths were all around us. But the friend who emailed me *had* survived, recurrence-free, for years, and so had dozens more people we knew. We were lifetimes—and saved lives—away from the warzone of 1975.

My friend had sent me this twenty-first-century metaphor instead of his thoughts and prayers, and I was grateful I wasn't barraged with prayers from my sensible, godless friends, but the message led me to wondering. "Do you remember when Christopher Hitchens got can-cer," I asked James as I lowered the shades, getting ready for bed, "and people who'd criticized his atheism asked if he was going to start be-lieving in God? Do you think this will turn us into believers?"

A pause. But the longer it went on, the more I feared his answer. "It would be a miracle," he said finally, with Jamesian irony. "What do you think?"

"Same." I nodded and switched off the light, which was my answer to another question that had been rattling around in my closet of fears: now that I had my diagnosis, would I do a Sontag and sleep with the lights on? Not tonight.

Not yet anyway.

Maybe It Was the Krazy Glue

That first day turned out to be the template for many to come: terrors and comforts flew back and forth like tennis balls at Wimbledon. Not to mention all the mysteries of the body to contend with. And so many one-way conversations we engaged in, my body and I. How many carcinogens had I consumed over the years—and how could I measure them? Had hair dye made me sick, or too much sugar, or was it that Krazy Glue I once used to repair a piece of pottery, then soaked my fingers in bleach to remove it? I regretted doing both seconds later, but the poisons were already seeping into my bloodstream. The body did not answer. Unless you're a smoker who gets lung cancer or you've spent years in a Monsanto plant, there's just radio silence. And maybe cancer behavior is no match for cancer genes, for the ordinary process of aging, the random arrow of bad luck that lands on the bull's eye that is the body. All of my valiant, hypochondriacal efforts to keep carcinogens from seeping into my bloodstream, including organic dental floss—I was *really* teed off about that—had been for the birds.

Beyond the unrequited conversations, I had the practical considerations of what to do with my eight essay clients and all the parents who called and emailed me almost every day wanting my help for their kids. I didn't have a colleague or anyone to send them to. The work is my relationship with the kids, built up over many weeks and sometimes months, and they were engaged in a complex project: discovering how to write about their lives, their interests, their ambitions. If I saw the doctor on October 4, how soon after that might treatments start? How debilitating would they be? Could I fake being OK while talking to people on Skype?

As I made coffee the morning after day number one, remembering

Prufrock "measuring out my life in coffee spoons," I decided that in the two weeks before my appointment, I would schedule extra sessions with students and delicately push them to work harder and faster. I would say no to any new clients who called. I would try not to think about the money I would not make, the money the doctor and the treatments would cost, the bills the insurance company would not pay. The plot of the story was whether I would survive my illness. The subplot was whether I could afford it.

Varieties of Religious Experience

Once I was diagnosed, I made two big changes: I stopped touching the hinge of my underarm, going from fifty feels a day to zero. And I stopped looking up anything online or between the covers of books on the subject of this disease. There was much I didn't know about my condition, notably what "stage" I was at, but I knew I couldn't find the answer anywhere but from a PET scan.

I was convinced that a significant number of my five hundred to seven hundred lymph nodes were malignant because I felt crappy in a way I never had before, not for an hour or a day at a time but every day. My legs and forehead itched, and I had a low-grade fever, shortness of breath, and bizarre aches and pains in my back and shoulders. My bones actually hurt, which I did not think was possible unless they had been broken or hit. The disease had spread to my organs and bone marrow—the months of waiting convinced me. There was no point in gathering more information, and there was this: I might scroll down my computer screen or turn the page of a book and run into a sea of statistics—one of which would be hard to unsee: how long I was likely to live.

I knew which variables influence the numbers. Worse outcomes over sixty, which I was, by a few years. Worse outcomes with lumps on both sides of the body. I could feel them only on my right side, but who knew what vipers might be lurking on my left? And worse outcomes if there are lumps around the clavicle. From what I could feel, I was home free on that one. The dreaded PET scan would see clear inside me, a glass-bottom boat peering into my cells, my organs, and my soul, lighting up wherever an outsize cluster of cells appears. The scan would look like a slice of Swiss cheese.

My sister's repertoire changed too. She never again mentioned Buddhist chanting and instead moved into high gear, finding me a wig for the chemo treatments that she was certain would follow. Her work as a beloved pediatric physical therapist with an extreme sect of Hasidic Jews, where all the women wear wigs, put her in touch with people who buy and sell a lot of headgear. Nancy took care of their children—and they would take care of Nancy's sister. Her seamless transition from Buddhist chanter to I Can Get it For You Wholesale wig broker was a beam of lightness and a lesson in the adaptability of religion through the ages.

I Got Sick Then I Got Better

Within days, Nancy learned that gray wigs made of real hair don't exist because when gray hair is cut, it turns yellow. Gray wigs have to be made of synthetic material, and my sister's source knew a place that sold them in midtown Manhattan. But there was a catch: the autumn Jewish holidays, which go on for weeks, were coming up, and the shop would be closed starting any day. I had to hurry or be shut out for a long time.

The night before my appointment, I broke my No Information policy and did some research online about the world of wigs. I figured I was safe. Watching wig videos, I was sure I wouldn't stumble onto information on how many years I had left to live. But I never imagined that watching a video about writer Jenny Allen's visit to a high-end wig store on Columbus Circle—from her show, *I Got Sick Then I Got Better*—would bring me a mantra that soothed me as Nancy's Tibetan chanting soothed her. The title leapt into my lap and curled up there like a purring cat. I said it to myself whenever I panicked about what would happen to me: *I Got Sick Then I Got Better*. Just saying it reminded me that if this happened to Jenny Allen—who had ovarian cancer—it just might happen to me too.

Cancer Hats

By appointment only, the wig store, on the fourth floor of a dingy office building in the West 30s, resembled a dingy beauty salon with no customers: a few raised swivel chairs and corresponding mirrors and shelves packed with wigs perched on mannequin heads. That day, the prospect of having no hair was abstract because I didn't know how soon I would need the wig. And winter was coming, so whenever it was that my hair fell out, I could cover my bald head with a hat and hide my condition from outsiders. Another benefit of working at home: if you go chemo-bald, it's easier to hide—the baldness and the illness, which I was determined to do with everyone outside my immediate circle.

"I know women who are more upset about losing their hair than they are about having cancer," said a doctor friend who specializes in breast cancer.

I was not one of them. I find the issues around hair and identity fascinating—hair as a cultural signifier, hair as a combat zone between mothers and daughters—but my own hair is not high on my list of obsessions. The energetic young woman in the shop that day brought me two gray wigs to try on. They matched my salt and pepper hair and one was more palatable than the other, short and layered with bangs—not my grandmother's shellacked curls and blue-tinted gray. I said almost nothing as I tried them, and she asked no nosy questions. Between us there were no beauty-salon intimacies, though I was sitting in a chair that probably elicited rivers of them. She must have known how to read people sitting in those hot seats, and she could read that I was in no mood either to chat or to confide.

At the checkout counter was an assortment of stretchy hats, some decorated with mini-scarves. I bought three—*Live it up*, I said under my breath—and thought of them as my "cancer hats," but only to myself, because I could not bear to say the word out loud to anyone. As I walked west to the subway, I discovered a vast store and another right beside it that I could see through the windows sold only ribbons. I must have come upon New York's ribbon district, an offshoot of the garment district. Through a window I saw only ribbons—thousands of them stacked on towering wooden shelves: waves of silk, lace, cotton, velvet, polka dots, stripes, hearts, flowers—no end to the patterns, colors, and textures.

When I entered the store, my whole being swelled with the profusion of colors and textures and the old-fashioned charm of the place. The shelves were ancient wood, nicked, worn, and jammed with ribbons wrapped around spools and bobbins, ribbons piled up, down, and sideways, like used books jam-packed into the shelves of the Strand, each book a different size with a different spine. The place was abuzz with women examining, comparing, measuring against rulers embedded in tables, and asking clerks to scissor their selections. I wished I could do clever things with needle and thread or whatever people do with these miles of ribbons, but what? I did not see trimming curtains or decorating wastebaskets in my future.

When I spotted a stack of ribbons that were wide, bright strips of silk, I knew: I would replace the dreary scarves on my cancer hats, just the thought of which made me absurdly happy. Even with cancer, a word I could barely whisper to myself, I was capable of feeling this outsized pleasure over something as inconsequential as ribbons. They brought me something that had been in short supply for many months.

Another mantra bubbled up: *Not every minute has to be misery.* I spent forty-seven dollars, which was a small price to pay for all this joy.

When Toni Morrison's House Burned Down

I had heard decades earlier that after Toni Morrison's country house burned down in 1993, she only wanted to talk to people whose houses had burned down. I was baffled. I thought I understood how dramatic the event was, but I also thought that her proscription was an affectation, the gesture of a diva. But when my own house—the house of health—was on fire, I got it. Got it because I had a version of her edict myself. I wanted most to talk to people who had faced what I was facing because I needed to know that I too might survive. Yet I had no interest in a support group. That would be too many people whose houses were on fire. Some of them wouldn't make it, and I knew I would hear stories about those in the group who hadn't made it—and I preferred solitary confinement to that.

It was all I could do to get from one day to the next with some semblance of normalcy as I waited. And waited. And waited some more. A semblance of normalcy because I had to be on my game as I worked intensively with four or five students a day, often for six hours in a row, and I was in a relationship. It was with a man who is kind, sensitive, and undemanding, one who listened whenever I wanted to talk about what I was going through, but who—and who can blame him?—did not want to hear me express my fear every time I opened my mouth. I did not have to pretend I felt fine, but I felt an obligation to James, to our daily life, to the maintenance of my wobbly equilibrium, to have more to offer than a playlist of thirty-seven songs about terror.

"I don't want to tell James how terrible I'm feeling," I said to my friend Dan on the phone. "I ache all over. I'm short of breath."

"You think he doesn't know?" Dan asked.

"Of course he knows I'm afraid, but . . ." I couldn't finish the sentence. I just knew I did not want to report to him every new fear, every new symptom. Our primary topic of conversation was now my health, with forays into what he was teaching. We couldn't make plans for next week or next month. And though I did not sleep with the lights on, I sometimes woke up in the middle of the night crying. James was the soundest sleeper on planet Earth, but now he'd wake up within seconds and reach for me. He knew all he needed to know.

As I write this now, I wonder why the encouraging words about my lymphoma being "treatable" didn't calm me right down. I have to remind myself that I had read enough by then—though I was no longer reading about it anymore—to know it was more complicated than that. And that it was easy for doctors to say things that Huck Finn would call "stretchers." The statement "I think this is curable" covered a multitude of possibilities, including that it was not.

And as I tell this story now, it's shaded by what we would soon find out. The case was more complicated than we could have imagined.

On Silence

Silence is not just the absence of sound.

Cancer is not contagious, though it has so many dimensions—those that attach to people around the patient and those that bear down on us if we are the patient—it sometimes feels as though it's contagious. There are better and worse kinds, cancer *back then* and cancer *now*. There are so many ways and places it can appear and re-appear and so much uncertainty about outcomes, it might be one of the scariest words in the language.

Unlike the charged words *mother*, *money*, and *marriage*, which stutterers often stumble over, for most of its history, cancer has been synonymous with death, and in that way, it is too much like another scary "m" word, *murder*, though there is far more cancer in this world than murder. It is also similar to *divorce*, which is not contagious either, but when it comes too close—because of a friend or loved one—it is a billboard-size reminder that we are all vulnerable. Memento mori. It's not *way out there*, it's *right here*. One day you're fine, and the next day your husband texts you that he's leaving or you finally summon the courage to leave him, and his world shatters. And within six months, three other couples you know split up. Or at the moment you're marveling at how happy you are, you touch a body part you don't usually touch and *thwack!*

I told no one in my building I was sick, including the people whose front door was three feet from mine, told few relatives, and because I was not in touch with them when this began, I never told a number of close friends—and still have not.

On the subject of not telling friends, the loquacious Nora Ephron was the Zen master of silence and secrecy about her leukemia. Her approach was the opposite of the photo and message I once found on Facebook: a glaring close-up of a gruesomely reddened eyeball, with the poster asking for advice on the treatment she needed. I much prefer the ways of solitary sufferers, though my own reticence was nowhere near the total blackout Nora engineered about her illness. In *Everything Is Copy*, the documentary her son Jacob Bernstein made about her, we hear one of her closest friends describe what she did not know would be their last lunch. Nora ordered dessert, which she never did, and wanted to take a cab home—three blocks—and she was hospitalized and gone a short time later, never having said *a word*. I did no such thing to *most* of my closest friends, but I understood the urge not to broadcast.

In 2012, I had emailed Nora, inviting her to be part of the anthology I planned to edit of women writing about a favorite gift from their mothers. "Your book sounds great," she wrote, "and I will certainly buy it. But I have written endlessly about my mother and I don't have another thing to say about her." Sixteen months later, she died, and soon after, I read a piece by Frank Rich about his not knowing she had been sick and wondering if she had not considered him such a close friend after all, though he'd always thought of *her* as a close friend. If they were as close as he always thought, didn't that mean she would have confided a terminal diagnosis?

Is the answer behind Curtain Number One, Two, or Three?

"Don't Ask Me How I Am"

"You can do this however you want," Zanti told me many times. "It's your choice." You can choose to spread the news with photos and posts on Facebook or you can choose silence, exile, and cunning. You can do a full Nora, Nora lite, Toni Morrison's diva delight, or any variation you dream up.

One reason Nora kept quiet was because it would have been difficult for her to make her last movie, *Julie and Julia*, if the moneymen had known she was so sick. On a much smaller scale, I was determined not to let any of the parents or kids I worked with know what was going on because I knew that, in their shoes, I would have dropped me in an instant. There was too much at stake to count on someone who might be preoccupied *and* had a sketchy future.

I kept the news from my only remaining aunt and uncle, whose three adult children have muscular dystrophy, and whose oldest was, at the time I was sick, being treated for the nonsmoking kind of lung cancer. They had enough *tsuris* for many lifetimes. *As long as you're healthy*, is my aunt's reflexive comment. How could I tell her I wasn't? *I'm fine!* I chirped on the phone, extra loud.

Cancer is not contagious any more than divorce is, but they are both bad news that spooks other people, and there can be around both a sense of personal responsibility, failure, and shame. The marriage failed, the body failed, and I'm sure it was my fault.

To the extent I was reticent, my reticence surprised me because I grew up being told that if I talk about my feelings, I'll feel better. I know of a thousand situations in which that's true, and aren't my feelings my bread and butter as a writer? Aren't they the water I swim in when I'm not writing, when I'm merely telling a story, listening to the stories of friends and family and students I work with? But when it came to sharing the sea of emotions in which I was treading water, there were long periods when I stopped talking. When I hid behind a wall. When I didn't have the words or the energy or the inclination to answer the most basic question on everyone's lips: "How are you?"

It seemed ridiculous to say *fine* but just as ridiculous to go into a metaphysical explanation of what it feels like to be in a profound state of limbo. Once my treatment began, I sent a long email to a group of friends and closed with: "Please don't ask me any version of how I am or how I'm doing." I knew that sounded harsh, so I added: "Just send book and movie and TV recommendations." They arrived in abundance.

If cancer was, even in my fantasies, the new puberty, it came with much of puberty's disorientation and shape-shifting: This new body was freaky—and most definitely not my friend. Like the changes of puberty, cancer and its treatments brought a boatload of surprises, nearly all of them—except some of the weight loss—unwelcome. Though I fleetingly heard Sontag's voice pressing me not to metaphorize cancer, it *is* literally an invasion, things growing inside us that don't belong, that threaten our survival, *that we can't control*—and this is where the matter of my silence comes in.

I had many reasons not to want to talk about this icy sea, but the one that took longest to understand was that my silence was the only element in this drama that I could control. My silence was a desperate power grab the way not eating is a power grab for the anorexic. And my silence was suppressed, inchoate anger at the universe that I knew it would have been pointless for me to express.

The Matter of Metaphors

When there's a cure, cancer will no longer inspire metaphors. When there's a cure, doctors won't lie and fudge and pretend you're fine and speak to you in code because they hate telling patients bad news. You'll get a diagnosis without drama and go for treatment like you go for a flu shot. Until then, what's wrong with a metaphor or two?

Cancer is swimming in the ocean when the ocean floor drops away and the rip tide has you. Cancer is dangling out of a helicopter by your ankle. Cancer is . . . write your own comparison in this space:

The Night Before

The good doctor's kindly receptionist told me to arrive at the office at ten o'clock the morning of October fourth and plan to spend the rest of the day there.

The night before the appointment, Emily came to stay with us again for several nights—she had rehearsals and an upcoming concert. Drifting from the dining room to our tiny kitchen, I told her a bit of what was going on—the big appointment tomorrow, my state of mind. She was tender and sweet, and now she was thirty years old and faced with a parent who had cancer. Standing at the kitchen counter, she turned to me and said, "You just have to fuck the cancer—just *fuck* it."

It was unlike her to talk that way to me, issuing proclamations, so certain and grown up. And she did not say "fuck" often in my presence, but it almost always made me think of an essay I wrote years ago about teaching her to swear when she was a young teenager, as a counterweight to her adolescent perfectionism, to the restraint and discipline she needed to play the violin the way she played. That night in our kitchen, she said, "Just *fuck it*," and turned away and said to the wall, "I'm going to cry."

I reached out and put my arms around her. "We can cry together." A hug, a few sniffles, nothing explosive but this moment of intimacy. And another mantra—I'd take anything on offer: *Fuck the cancer—just fuck it*. I liked the sound of it. I liked that it came from her.

A few minutes later at the dining room table, I told her I would stop eating sugar once the treatments got underway. "I've been reading all the anticancer diets, and they all said ix-nay with the sugar, even though the MSK website says that sugar has nothing to do with it. I know I have to stop, but it's hard."

"I'm reading a book," Emily said, "about a woman with a rare form of cancer, and she created a high alkaline diet and no sugar."

"But how will I survive without chocolate chip cookies?"

"Don't think about what you can't eat. Think about what you can. You can make cookies with dates." A pause. "I don't mean to tell you what to do." She was used to my being the one who told her what to do—though much less often than when she was younger.

"Tell me," I implored her now. "It's fine. Tell me anything."

I'm not sure she told me everything on her mind, any more than I told her everything on mine. I had never told her how I had imagined my later years would unfold, that I assumed I would outlive both her parents, as I have many relatives who lived well into their nineties and one into her early one hundreds. And now I didn't tell her that I had to reimagine my future, and that I might join her Aunt Janet in the family's Women Who Die Young series—though it had to have been on everyone's mind.

Deena's mantra was never far from my thoughts. *Cancer will make you humble. And you will learn something from it.*

Humility was coming easily to me—I mean, there's not much to it when you're on your way to the oncologist's office for the entire day. But as far as what I would learn—what exactly was I on the lookout for?

The Gene

The doctor made an announcement moments after we sat down in his office, before he examined me: "You are positive for a gene that makes you less responsive to the chemo."

He was a big, not-quite-burly man, and every surface of his small office was crammed with diplomas, plaques, medical *tchotchkes*, and stacks of manila patient files. His pathologists had done genetic testing on the slides he'd requested—and discovered the positive gene.

"There are two kinds of chemo I would use with this. The second has to be administered in the hospital. Five days, every three weeks, six times. There's no data on how effective the chemo is with this gene, but that's my recommendation right now." He said the name of the gene, and James wrote it in the notebook on his lap, the temperature in the room plummeting with this news.

"I might add a drug that's used to treat leukemia," he offered, "though that's not what you have. It can counteract the effects of the gene." I would learn that the drug costs ten thousand dollars a bottle, a bottle lasts for a month, and because I didn't have leukemia, my insurance might not pay for it. And thirty nights in the hospital mainlining chemo would turn me into a cancer cadaver. I would not be able to work, pay for the health insurance, or pay for the drugs. I would have to raid my retirement account or borrow money or organize a GoFundMe campaign, or all three. I would shrivel up and become a bald bag of bones. Please don't ask me how I am.

Minutes later, in the tiny exam room, the doctor said, "Your blood pressure is *very* high," and snapped off the Velcro sleeve around my arm.

I could barely speak. James sat on a straight-backed chair taking notes, not looking up. The words "It's usually low" crept out of my mouth.

Moments later, back in his office, he found an important piece of paper on his desk: the results of my PET scan, which had not been put into my file. An old-fashioned doctor in an old-fashioned office where someone had long ago tossed out a memo about switching over to computers for patient records. All four doctors still used manila files, towering, dog-eared stacks on every desk and every surface in the reception cubicle. The PET scan report, which had wandered into the office from God knows where, contained news.

"The only evidence of disease in your body is in the axilla," the doctor announced. Latin for armpit. "There's nothing else anywhere. Instead of six times in the hospital, you'll only need three times." Fifteen days, not thirty.

A reprieve. A little bit better than I was twenty minutes ago, but how exactly to measure emotions when they are so extreme? Fifteen days of chemo, 24/7, was now the good news. I sent emails to friends when I had good news. I did not send any emails about this gene, though I told Zanti that afternoon when we got home, told her the name of the gene—and immediately regretted it. She would Google it and learn the awful truth about my life expectancy. The Internet might as well have posted the date of my death for the fear it stirred up in me.

And James would Google it too and know my grim fate, if he didn't already, the dark truth about my future—and his own. I was nauseated with fright. "I have to tell you something," I told James as we sat in the living room that night. "Please don't Google the gene. I told Zanti, and now I regret it."

He paused before saying, "OK." Or maybe he had already Googled it?

"Do you promise?" I myself had not looked it up—and would not. He nodded.

"I don't want you to know something awful about me, because I don't want to know it myself. And don't tell Emily."

"OK."

"If you Google it, it will be a terrible betrayal. Like sleeping with someone else."

"I won't. I promise."

How crazy was I in those moments?

I was cancer crazy. I was scared to death, and based on the news about this gene, I had every reason to be.

One Hundred Flowers

Early the next morning, I returned alone to the doctor's office, to an-other of the small exam rooms that line a long hallway, for a bone bi-opsy, to see if the cancer had penetrated my bones. It would explain why I had so much pain when I pressed on my shoulders and my shins.

"The doctor will be here in a few minutes," said the women who'd walked me back there and closed the door behind her. The exam room was tiny, the furnishings and equipment felt like 1970, or maybe 1950, though the stacks of magazines—*Harper's Bazaar, The Econo-mist,* and *Living with Cancer*—were up to date. The cover story, a smiling woman and the banner "I'm Having the Time of My Life!" made me wince and flip to the next. I wanted fantasies, luxury, air-brushed stories of celebrity dwellings, not faux happy people making the most of their rotten luck, because I was one of them now. Give me ads for infinity swimming pools and houses made of glass overlook-ing turquoise waters. The time of her life? What kind of feel-good-New-Age crap was that? Even the Girl Scouts looked good next to this team-I-didn't-want-to-join.

A knock on the door and then it opened.

"Ready?" said the big but not-quite-burly doctor.

I lay face down on a padded table and braced for the stab to the back of my pelvic bone with a needle thick enough to push into the bone and suck out enough marrow to biopsy it. He shot my lower back with three or four rounds of Novocaine, and I soon began to chant silently: *Nam Myoho Renge Kyo, Nam Myoho Renge Kyo, Nam Myoho Renge Kyo, Nam Myoho Renge Kyo, Nam Myoho Renge Kyo,* as tears and snot filled my eyes and nose. Another template. Chanting through unbelievable pain. Chanting through this dive into dread my life had taken.

It was a job for a young man, a carpenter, a guy with a drill: pushing a needle into human bone. *Nam Myoho Renge Kyo, Nam Myoho Renge Kyo.*

"That's it," the doctor said. "Done!"

I was not sobbing, but he noticed the mess on my face and said, "You got good news yesterday! You're a stage one. That's great! And the pathologist told me there's another gene you *don't* have that could have made things *much* worse. You may not need to be in the hospital for all the treatments."

He had not given it a name until that moment—stage one! What hadn't he told me? All I'd heard yesterday was that I had this awful gene, and about the fifteen days of 24/7 chemo in the hospital.

"Given that," he said, "I suspect there's nothing in your bone marrow, but we'll know in a few days."

I wasn't having the time of my life just yet, but I walked out of the office with energy to burn and headed west, not sure of my destination until I was a few blocks from the Metropolitan Museum of Art. How would I manage all those days in the hospital? I imagined a jigsaw puzzle for when I got tired of reading and guessed I would find one in the museum's gift shop.

As I crossed the floor, I spotted a small book facing up on a display table, which turned out to be not a book but a box of postcards in the shape of a book: *100 Flowers*. On the spine was, "One Hundred Postcards from the Royal Horticultural Society." Antique botanical images on the back of which I could write my thoughts. Perfect! My one-hundred-day diary. I would somehow force this event—my new stage one illness—into those one hundred days and into this beautiful box.

And maybe I would actually send a few postcards—a lingering habit from the Sweet Days of Sending Postcards, which had only faded with the advent of email.

As I paid for the box, I remembered the story of poet Kaye Mc-Donough I had heard from writer friends when I lived in San Francisco after college. As she composed a play about Zelda Fitzgerald, in the time long before Post-It notes, she strung a clothesline across her writing room and used clothespins to hang her notes, like leaves on a tree, so she could walk among them. Wouldn't it be fun to do that in a corner of my dining room with my beautiful postcards? An indoor garden strung with antique botanicals on one side and, on the other, messages to myself and others and maybe my high-minded thoughts on the matter of my mortality.

And so it went, the seesaw of my moods. From hour to hour, they dove and soared, skated sometimes in long, elegant arcs of optimism and then skittered every which way in despair.

One Thousand Doctors on My Case

A few days later, the doctor's deep voice again on the phone. He called more often than my best friend did and even gave me his cell number without my asking. I might be cancer crazy with my husband, but I could put on a sanity show with the good doctor.

"I'm not sure about your treatments," he began. "I could put you in the hospital three times for five days each, but maybe I don't need to. Maybe you'll do just fine with the chemo that we can administer here, which takes a few hours every three weeks. There's no data on how best to deal with this gene of yours, so I'm going to survey my colleagues. We're having our annual meeting—a thousand doctors—the week after next, and I'm going to ask them what they would do with you."

"Are you going to make an announcement?" A thousand faces, a thousand arms popping up to vote yes or no on my future. Would I become a case study? Would my treatment plan really come down to counting the votes of strangers in a Hilton ballroom?

"No." The doctor's kindly, mild chuckle. "That's not how it's done. I talk to them privately."

I felt fleeting disappointment that I would not get the benefit of a thousand opinions. But if I was going to die, could I at least become a study in something? "Do other people not have the gene?" I ventured.

"Yes, but it usually turns positive after treatment, not before treatment starts. And it spooks me."

The word reverberated like a tuning fork. It spooked me too, and it spooked me even more that *he* was spooked. I'd gone from doctors who were afraid to tell me I might have cancer to a doctor so candid about my condition that the two of us might end up on suicide watch with the combined total of our fears about what lay ahead.

Should I have asked him more questions? Should I have gone full Deena and pressed him on details, possibilities, odds and ends? How could I? I was frozen in place. And he'd settled it. *He* was spooked. And he was going to take a vote. Or whatever he was going to do with the thousand doctors.

The seesaw of emotions sometimes goes sideways as well as up and down.

Fortunately, I couldn't perseverate on the matter every waking minute because I had six or eight high school students who needed practical help with their college application essays, and the work, going from word to word and line to line on a shared Google Doc, demanded my full attention. In fact, it was the only activity that shut off my anxiety engine for hours at a time, but I tensed up when we got to the end of each session and I had to schedule our next meeting. When would treatments begin—and would I do them in the doctor's office or in a hospital? The first college applications were due in three weeks, and I booked appointments with students five to seven days in advance. I toyed with saying to them, "Someone in my family is sick and may have to go to the hospital, and I'll be busy with that for a while." While I toyed, I scheduled sessions sooner, and kids were happy getting their essays done more quickly.

If I told them what was wrong, the news could end up online, in a review on Yelp, or in a Facebook comment that would never go away. It sounds far-fetched, but that doesn't mean it wouldn't happen. The stakes were sky-high for all of us.

Cancer and Cancer Stories

There are three kinds of cancers: Terminal, Curable, The Rest of Them.

Which means that there are at least three kinds of cancer stories to write and, on the other end, to read.

I began writing mine early in what I resist calling "my cancer journey," but could not get far because the story was evolving. The story, you might say, was *still being written*—but not by me. I could describe what had happened, but my uncertain future made it impossible to find a tone, a voice, a relationship to the material. Writers with a terminal diagnosis, those lucky so-and-so's, have a built-in source of energy to power what they write. They have an antagonist—mortality—and a ticking clock. It's their last chance to have the last word.

I had not been given a dire diagnosis, so I wrote my story, this story, for the longest time without that manic energy, but without any other identifiable texture or tone. It was flat, and I was frustrated, and my frustration went on and on. If only, I sometimes caught myself saying, If only I had a terminal diagnosis, I'd know exactly how to write this.

But I am jumping ahead.

Cancer Is a Power Struggle

On one of those nights as I waited to start my treatment and practiced saying, with a straight face, "Someone in my family is sick and may have to be in the hospital soon," my sister called with a pronouncement. Seconds after "hello," she said, "I'll shave my head in solidarity." I was briefly speechless and rushed in with, "No, that's fine! You don't have to do that!" I was too stunned to be as touched as I came to be. She would shave the head of hair that meant so much to her? Really? Long hair that she straightens, colors, highlights, and makes sure always looks great? It would take years to grow back! "That's not necessary," I added.

I was in a mild state of shock. We did not come from a family of activists who made dramatic sacrifices. No hunger strikes, no chaining ourselves to fences surrounding nuclear power plants. We'd had enough problems growing up without adding "suffering in solidarity" to our repertoire.

"I didn't think you'd want me to," she admitted.

"But thank you."

Within moments, I remembered the true story that Deborah Hofmann tells in her essay in *Me, My Hair and I*. Before her chemo treatments, her husband suggested what Nancy had, but with an added twist: husband and wife got their heads shaved *together* at the local salon. It was a heartwarming, girl-gotta-great-husband story, but when it was my turn up at bat, I wanted no announcements, no grand gestures, no group activities, nothing but to slink away in solitude, even after Emily told me that she thought bald-headed women look cool. In the days and weeks that followed, Nancy asked me repeatedly what I would do to get ready for my hair falling out, which the doctor said would start about two weeks after the chemo began, whenever that was.

"If you cut it short," Nancy suggested, "when it comes out, it'll be easier to deal with."

"OK." I had no plans to cut it.

"If you consult a hairdresser," Nancy said, "maybe they'll have some ideas for how to make it happen more smoothly."

"OK." I was not going to consult anyone or look up ideas online. Doing anything at all was like rearranging the deck chairs on the *Titanic*. Why spend a minute fussing over hair that's going to fall out? Nothing I did would make me less bald. Nancy's suggestions were what she imagined she would do, faced with losing her hair.

Yet all this time later, I understand two things: that my sister's offer to cut off her hair in solidarity was a love letter to me—and our family was not big on those either—and that my refusal to make preparations for losing my hair *was* my plan. It seems I was a bit more vain than I had been willing to admit: I was going to hang onto every goddam strand until it quit me.

Sontag 2.0: *Cancer is a power struggle. When it's not an outright war.*

Living with Cancer

The next time the doctor called was to report that my first round of chemo would mean five days in the hospital. Soon after, he would attend the meeting of a thousand doctors and query them: should I do the remainder in five-day hospital sprints or what I called chemo-al-fresco, sitting in one of those little exam rooms in his office, passing the time reading back issues of *Vogue* and *Living with Cancer*?

"What day will I go to the hospital?" I asked.

"We never know. You're on a list, and when a bed is free, they call you, the night before or the morning of."

What? This sounded more like going to the ER. *Someone in my family is sick and has to go to the hospital, but we're not sure when?*

I had already begun saying a version of it to my clients. "Oh, by the way," I'd begin. "I may not be able to meet with you next week. Things are still up in the air."

Plenty was up in the air while I hovered out on the ledge, but one certainty was a book I would take with me to the hospital, Evelyn's gift of *Miss Pettigrew Lives for a Day* by Winifred Watson, because of the inscription she had written on the frontispiece: "This is the only 'feel-good' book that ever really made me feel good—so in your time of need, I hope it works for you."

Where Had I Been All My Life?

It was a case of cancer for dummies.

I have dozens of friends and a few relatives who've had cancer, but I had no clue where or how this thing called chemo happened. When I heard mine would go down in a hospital, I imagined a dreary double room with a roommate behind a curtain suffering her own private ailment while I lay in bed with an IV on a pole by my side. I assumed I'd be largely ignored from one hour to the next. It would be an ordeal to get a nurse to come in, as it had been the times my mother had been hospitalized. And because I was going to be there for five nights, I splurged and bought an oversized Indian silk tunic with a bold black and white design and baggy sleeves so there would be room for the IV. I was thinking of everything!

But I knew absolutely nothing.

When the woman called from the hospital to tell me when to check in, I asked where I would be staying so I could tell visitors.

"The chemo ward, 10 North."

Chemo ward? I had no idea there was such a place and pictured a Spartan barracks-like room with two dozen beds, each inhabited by a wizened patient, more ancient opium den than twenty-first-century hospital.

Where had I been all my life?

And what do you bring to a hospital besides books, magazines, a jigsaw puzzle of a Matisse cutout, and a handful of botanical post-cards from my box of one hundred? Would I actually write cards to people and mail them? Unlikely. But I might scribble notes to myself, might fill up the blank sides with Thoughts from My Hospital Room.

When my dearest friend Zanti offered to come to New York from hundreds of miles away and spend her days with me in the hospital because she knew how nervous I was, it was easy to say, "No, not necessary," but hard to believe how much she was willing to do for me. Didn't she know that I could do this on my own? Hadn't she known me long enough—more than four decades—to know that I complained and emoted, but I did what needed to be done? Yet if it had been Zanti going to the hospital with cancer and being as afraid as I was, I'm sure I would have offered the same. And pretty sure she would have said what I did: that she could handle it by herself.

The Chemo Ward

The silver letters over the double doors leading from 10 Central to 10 North said, "Medical Oncology." Inside the doors was a hallway flanked by patient rooms and leading to a broad nurses' station, with seats for five or six people, overlooking a lounge area and a huge window with a view of the northern skyline. Many of the buildings I could see were part of the hospital complex, alongside a swath of the raging brown waters of the East River and Queens in the dreary distance. Not a beautiful sight, but a dramatic, appropriate one—severe, cold, utterly serious. I was assigned a large square corner room right off the nurses' station with two huge windows looking north and west. My corner of the room had the two windows, while my roommate, in the other corner, lay hidden behind curtains on two sides. She had privacy back there but no window, no light but the fluorescent. I had hit the real estate jackpot. And a short time later, the health jackpot too, when the doctor called. "Your bone marrow is clean," he said.

"No disease." I texted James the good news, which he would read when he finished teaching that day.

Sunlight poured in, and as I took up residence in the armchair near my bed, I thought again of Nora Ephron. I knew she had been treated and had died in this building. One of the last shots in *Everything Is Copy* is the hospital's distinctive towers, the elongated, pointy, Gothic-style windows—the hospital as cathedral. I wanted to know what room she'd been in, though it seemed ghoulish to ask, grotesquely gossipy—and I knew I wouldn't get an answer. And there were no assurances I would not one day meet the same fate in the very same place. But at the moment, the connection was strangely reassuring. It meant that, like Nora Ephron, I was getting the best possible care, which was, in itself, startling.

As a full-time, full-blown hypochondriac, I had worried all my adult life about what would become of me if I ever "became sick," and for that reason spent an inordinate amount of time and money making sure I had good health insurance, even as a struggling writer. I had read so many articles about people with cancer going bankrupt, even those with insurance, that even in the hospital with my excellent coverage, I went over my list of prosperous friends and relatives whom I might have to ask for money later on, if this got out of hand, if I was faced with something drastic. How long was the list? Would I ask for a specific amount or *pay what you wish?* I composed many drafts of these letters in my head.

But worry wasn't the dominant chord on 10 North. From my armchair, I could see the nurses' station a few feet outside my door and, when I turned my head, a slice of the East River and a lot of sky. Streams of people came and went doing their jobs, all remarkably kind and efficient. A team of nurses appeared and performed an elaborate procedure to insert a peripherally inserted central catheter, or

PICC line, into a vein in my upper arm so that an assortment of plastic tubes and catheters could be attached to it and the chemo could do its dripping.

So much for the beautiful black and white silk tunic for my "hospital stay." My upper arm was hospital property, the conduit for the cure, and my wardrobe was a hospital gown with easy access to every inch of my body. I had imagined that I would chat with my roommate, maybe even get to know her, but I did not feel comfortable even introducing myself to her, nor she to me, though when she emerged to use the bathroom, we sometimes nodded at each other. It dawned on me that we were like people in lockup or prison, a place no one wanted to be, a place we'd landed because of serious troubles. The last thing we wanted to do was make small talk, and the second-to-last was big talk, to ask or be asked: "What are you in for?"

Miss Pettigrew on 10 North

I had brought a pile of old *New Yorkers* and a few books, and soon I was ensconced in the armchair, devouring *Miss Pettigrew Lives for a Day*, smiling, sometimes laughing out loud. Evelyn was entirely right—it did make me feel good, and by the end of the first night, the first bag of chemo having already dripped into my bloodstream. I was buffeted ever so gently by a series of surprises:

I could actually concentrate on this otherworldly English novel about a reserved governess sent out on a job by an agency but sent to the wrong address—the home of a sexual libertine whose pajamed lover is just getting up when she arrives. No children to care for, but there is a full day of lessons to learn about the thrilling, dangerous ways of men and women. Hour by hour, Miss Pettigrew sloughs off layers of stodginess and eventually her chastity. By day's end, she's a bold adventuress ready for love, "brimming with authority and assurance. . . . She thought scornfully of her former timid self. A futile creature! Fear! Had she once known fear? Impossible."

In my room on 10 North, I did not feel grand or brimming with authority and assurance. But after four solid months of fear—on this, Miss P. and I were soulmates—and all the doctors who said, "Chill out" while my tumors and my terror grew, I was chill enough to relish a book as far from the circumstances of my life as a book could be.

In my corner room, with three catheters hanging from a hole in my upper arm like keys on a keychain, I was calmer than I had been since the moment on June ninth when I first felt the lump.

Postcard #1

I am happy I have no one to talk to.

I am happy to be alone.

I am happy to be in the hospital, to get three meals a day that I order from a long menu and are not the hospital mush I was expecting.

I am just plain happy because, for the first time in more than four months, I am where I belong, and I'm being taken care of.

Surprise of surprises, I am happy in the chemo ward.

Walking My Way to Recovery

One of the drugs in the chemo cocktail is the steroid prednisone, which suppresses nausea. A side effect makes you feel you can hit a ball at ninety-five miles an hour out of Yankee Stadium, and maybe you can. "The steroids might make you manic," said the shrink I'd been seeing. "You might have ideas for ten books."

"That doesn't sound so bad." Bring them on! Line up those meds on my laptop.

Once the stuff was coursing through my veins, I waited for the mania. Waited and waited but nothing. Not even a flutter. How could that be? A day later, I figured it out: I'd been down so long, the steroids just got me back to zero, to the cheerful person I used to be.

During the days, the hallways were mobbed with people, carts, and machines on wheels. At night, the place was eerily quiet, and I hit the road. I walked up and down the halls for exercise, pulling my IV pole, wearing nothing more than a hospital gown thirteen sizes too big. The IV pole carried a heavy bag of poisonous liquid that was attempting to slay the cancer cells multiplying inside me. Would it work—or would I be the guy in the TV commercial for a cancer center whose lymphoma didn't respond to chemo and he needed something else—was it a bone marrow transplant?—to crush these overactive cells? Susan Sontag be damned: this was armed combat at the cellular level, and it was unclear which side would prevail.

Mostly, though, I didn't think about doing battle as I walked night after night from 10 North to 10 Central to 10 South and around again and again, past patient rooms, rooms labeled "Negative Pressure Room," past colorful signs posted high on the walls every ten or fifteen feet that said: "WALK YOUR WAY TO RECOVERY!" Past long counters lined with nurses and technicians sitting at computers and past bold, colorful, abstract works of art on the walls, mostly signed prints, not framed posters, that gave me immense pleasure. That made me stop and study the play of color and shape and the texture of the paper, that made me remember James' and my second date in an art gallery in what was then the Meatpacking District, before its complete gentrification. We took a creaky, creepy service elevator to a fourth-floor warren of sun-filled rooms and found that we both loved paintings by Cy Twombly. And I thought of my mother, who all her life made art—drawings, paintings, sculpture—including drawings with ink and pastel on the bathroom walls of the nursing home where she suffered from dementia. The day after she died, we held a small service for her, and I knew that the only way I would get through it was to force myself to think about her art instead of the difficult life she had lived, her art instead of the sadness and powerlessness that made me want to run from her, ensure that I would not be like her. But mostly on my night walks, I just felt happy about the abstract artwork on those walls. I did not have to tug my IV past schmaltzy landscapes or sentimental scenes of domestic life.

I was comforted by the thought that the artwork had been donated by artists who'd been patients there, and as my week went on, I decided that if I made artwork, I too would donate it to acknowledge how kind and competent everyone was who worked there. No grumblers, no malcontents, no sighs of displeasure at questions. They seemed like people who liked their jobs in the chemo ward, and that was as surprising to me as anything. Most of the hospital nurses I had encountered elsewhere seemed—miserable. And if they were, who could blame them? From all I knew, they were overworked, undervalued, and harassed by demanding patients, their families, and gropey old men. If they were unhappy on 10 North, they did not let on. And that counted for a lot, especially if I had to return for two more rounds, another ten or twelve days. I still didn't know.

If I had carried my iPhone, I could have counted the steps I walked back and forth on the leukemia ward and the bone marrow transplant ward and whatever other diseases were being treated—not battled, not vanquished—at my end of the hall. And if I had carried my iPhone, I could have taken notes for a radio essay on being in a chemo ward. Years before, I had done three or four on-air essays for National Public Radio, and as I walked my way to recovery one night, I thought: Why not a series on my "cancer journey," beginning here, on 10 North? Within seconds, I slammed the door on that idea. If the treatment didn't work, if my wonky gene was too much for the best doctor in the field, if the thousand doctors gave my doctor the wrong answer, if I really had to face my death and I was in the midst of recording "my journey," I would not want to talk about it on the radio.

I might not be walking my way to recovery after all.

Where Did She Come From?

Three days into the treatment, my roommate was discharged, and I looked forward to a day or two of single-room luxury. But overhead lights and many voices woke me at three o'clock Sunday morning. The metallic *swish* of the curtains being pulled back, the patient being moved from gurney to bed, the endless questions—in English and from somewhere behind the curtain, another voice repeating them in Spanish, the voice amplified on what sounded like a speaker phone. The fluorescent lights shone through my eyelids. The doctors spoke in their outside voices.

"What medications are you on?"

"Do you have any allergies?"

"We're going to be analyzing your blood work to see how we need to proceed."

"We may need to give you a blood transfusion."

"You have something called acute myeloid leukemia. It's a blood disease. It's important for you to know that you didn't do anything to cause it. It's not your fault. Do you understand?"

"Your husband can stay here, but all we have for him is this chair."

On and on they went for forty-five minutes, in two languages. I reached for my phone and some ear buds and punched a guided meditation podcast I had downloaded at Evelyn's suggestion, for times when Miss Pettigrew wasn't available. "This is the time to give yourself space and devote yourself to putting your worries and concerns away. It's time to bring happy thoughts and positive energy to the front of your mind. Before you begin your meditation . . ."

When I woke up a few hours later, one of the night nurses, a young man I was fond of, came to check my vitals. "Can I ask you something?" I said softly.

"Sure."

"Where did she come from at three a.m.? The emergency room?" I knew nearly everything else about her, but I really wanted to know how a person knows she has acute myeloid leukemia, because you never know when this information might matter.

"I'm sorry," he said, lowering his head toward mine. "I can't tell you."

Before long, she had a stream of visitors, what sometimes seemed like a dozen people speaking Spanish behind the curtains, and when I passed her bed, I saw she was a beautiful young woman with dark hair down to her waist, about the age of my stepdaughter.

Every medical exchange was broadcast in two languages. The doctors were kind and spoke slowly.

She would be in the hospital for a month.

Was she planning to have more children?

She and her husband had two now and they were hoping for more later on.

It was important for her to know that she might not be able to have more children, because of the treatment she was going to get. And her hair would fall out. Did she understand?

Si.

Did she have any questions?

Si. Would her children be able to visit her in the hospital?

The doctor wasn't sure. They would have to wait and find out how she does with the treatments.

When she got up to go to the bathroom and our eyes met, I would smile, and I could practically feel my heart cracking in my chest. Whatever happened to me, I felt I was the more fortunate of the two of us. I had lived many more decades without sickness than she had. I had had the time and good fortune to do more or less what I wanted with my life. I did not have to spend a month in the hospital. I did not have acute myeloid leukemia. I did not have small children who might lose their mother. I did not need a translator to talk to the doctor, and, for the time being, I had absurdly expensive health insurance that would pay most of the bill, and my hunch was that she did not.

When I told my sister about the commotion of this woman's arrival, she said, "Why can't you tell them to move you to another room?" Nancy didn't understand that I felt a kinship with her. She didn't understand that this is how it goes down on 10 North, in Medical Oncology, unless, for instance, you are Nora Ephron, who also had acute myeloid leukemia and, I'm quite sure, a private room. I've since learned that hers was on the thirteenth floor.

Housekeeping

Late on my last night in the hospital, James phoned to say how happy he was that I was coming home. And he had a question.

"What's that?"

"How does the Swiffer work?"

He had heard Nancy insist that we keep the apartment spotless, to make sure I was not exposed to germs in my immunocompromised state.

"You see the blue-green plastic box on the shelf? That's where the wet cloths are."

As I explained how to attach the cloths to the flat rubber end of the Swiffer, I had a flash of dreading to go home. I should want to leave the hospital, shouldn't I? Who wants to be in a hospital? But who wants to be sick at home and worried about every speck of dirt, about what to eat, about the contraption hanging out of my arm that pinched all the time, about taking a shower and getting it wet, and worried that tomorrow was the first day of the rest of my short, shitty life?

A Diamond as Big as the Ritz

When I departed the following morning, I didn't know whether I would be back for two more rounds of premium chemo on 10 North or chemo alfresco in the doctor's office. He still hadn't consulted his thousand colleagues, but at my appointment with him on my way home from the hospital, he examined me and gently pressed into my right axilla—which I hadn't touched for more than a month—and exclaimed, "Gone!"

The two remaining lymph nodes, the size of large jellybeans, had been crushed. The doctor was happy, but he didn't need to say that the spooky gene meant they could come back at any time. Instead, he handed me a bottle of the ten-thousand-dollar medicine prescribed for leukemia that he wanted me to take, another baseball bat to clobber the gene with. It was a sample or a patient's supply that wasn't needed—and now, in the palm of my hand, it was mine. I lodged it into a zippered pocket in my bag with trepidation. It could buy a two-carat diamond or a high-mileage used car.

"Take four pills a day," he said casually.

"For how long?"

"Three months."

No word yet on whether my insurance would pay for it, but a whopping thirty thousand dollars if not. And among the side effects: it might give me atrial fibrillation.

Next week, in a hotel ballroom, he would survey his thousand colleagues on the subject of my treatment.

Deena was right. I was humbled, nearly flattened, by all of this. And I was learning plenty. And all of it was for the birds.

Icarus on the Upper West Side

The chemo blues.

That's when the steroids wear off and the chemo reaches a certain threshold of maximum force and misery, though mine came with a bonus: a gift from a thousand lymphoma doctors who voted sixty to forty percent in favor of my having the remaining infusions in the office, not the hospital. Not a landslide but a clear victory, and I was elated. And happier still when the doctor told me to stop taking the ten-thousand-dollar leukemia pills after two weeks. Maybe he'd talked to his colleagues about that too? These triumphs made up for my hair falling from my scalp like autumn leaves from a maple tree. One morning when I clutched what was left, it was so stringy that, sitting on the couch without a mirror, I took a pair of scissors and cut all of it off in two snips right below my ears, my eyes widening in disbelief: it was like cutting a piece of paper.

The chemo blues were much worse than I had anticipated, and my metaphorical thinking revved up: a combination of flu minus fever plus jet lag. The key-ring-like catheter still dangled from my arm, pinching constantly. It had to be hermetically sealed before I could take a bath or shower; a drop of water could contaminate it. But my brain fog and energy weren't so bad that I couldn't gather my wits in small doses and work for a few hours a day with students on Skype, eventually donning one of the stretchy cancer hats decorated with a silk ribbon from the ribbon store. I preferred the hats to the wig, which was hot and uncomfortable. At moments I was slower than usual, I sometimes said to the kids, "Sorry, I'm feeling a little under the weather right now," which any adult, seeing the hat, would know how to translate. The students might have figured it out, but they didn't have the experience to ask about my situation—and they had more pressing matters on their minds.

In the big world outside my apartment, a new species of startling news was breaking every day and sending sparklers of distraction into my living room. Powerful men who had harassed, molested, or raped women in the workplace were losing their high-powered jobs in the wake of Ronan Farrow's explosive piece about Harvey Weinstein in the *New Yorker* from early October. It had seemed for a time that Farrow's piece would be the tale of one staggeringly awful man, but dozens more tumbled hard in the following weeks—including two old friends.

When I'd hear the front door open late in the day—James coming in from teaching and taking classes—I would shout out another man's name, and we'd bond while reviewing the new transgressions. We were suddenly privy to the tawdry secret lives of media and show biz darlings, and I'm sorry to say we were relieved we had this antidote for the anxiety that had gripped our household for so many months. As my cancer cells died, #MeToo was being born.

When the story got personal with news of our friends, our idle gossip took on weight, like a small boat taking on water. Who would be next? "Don't look at me," James answered, serious but joking, joking but serious.

And how were the two men we knew coping? They were friends of long standing, but what was the etiquette? Do you email them—oh, wait, the only email address you have is from work, and they've just been escorted out of the building by security. Do you call and say, "I'm sorry," or do you say, "*You did what?*" Another friend who was close to one of the men's wives finally sent her an "I'm-thinking-of-you-at-this-difficult-time" email. I knew the wife a little and had been in their apartment. I could visualize scenes of the fallout in the living room, the setting of parties packed with important people who lived in apartments every bit as lavish and tasteful as that one. I could imagine the wife's face, her anguish and rage at both the intimate betrayal and the social and economic plunge—Icarus on the Upper West Side. A hard landing. Do you stay or do you go? How do you look at him, talk to him, make sense of the lifelong partnership you thought you had, the children you raised together? "You did *what* to a woman who worked for you?"

"Are You Seeing Someone?"

Inside my apartment, I had my own secret life, turning away visitors, hiding from neighbors, watching as many HBO shows as I could during a free trial week. I binged on Season One of *Big Little Lies* and the Bernie Madoff miniseries, getting a crash course in the awful things men do, while I took inventory of my drug-addled existence on the couch. The chemo blues brought weakness, fatigue, depression, brain fog, stomach pain, ravenous hunger, constipation, scary weight loss, a long list of foods to be avoided—and I had a stove that didn't work. It hadn't worked for months and wouldn't anytime soon because Con Edison had to turn off the gas in the building while the owner repaired gas lines in 128 apartments. We made do with a microwave, with containers of yogurt, hardboiled eggs cooked in the electric kettle, huge salads, and grilled chicken and fish from Zabar's. James had lunch out almost every weekday with friends, my sister brought me containers of roasted vegetables, and a kind friend bought us an electric steamer.

Beyond my jerry-rigged kitchen, women kept speaking out, hot-shot men kept losing their jobs, and my first chemo treatment in the doctor's office led three weeks later to the second, the day before Thanksgiving. I was sylph-thin, my stomach hurt all the time, and I staggered into the office so obviously weak that the receptionist grabbed a wheelchair without my asking and pushed me to the exam room down the hall. Would the doctor dare give me another round of chemo in my feeble state? It was not possible.

They drew blood and the nurse attached a half dozen wires to my chest, monitoring my heart with a machine that cried out, "Made in 1960! Maybe 1965!" to see if I could withstand another round of chemo. Half an hour later, tears of exhaustion streaked my face as the doctor listened to my heart and lungs and pushed his fingers into places where wayward lymph nodes take hold, under my ribcage and into my lump-free armpit. While he worked, he kibitzed. His children, his wife, his patients. Some one-liners and sometimes shaggy dog stories about medical procedures gone awry that the doctor fixed, and one about a marriage gone sour that turned around after the bitter, overweight wife got cancer and lost so much weight that she became a happy sylph herself. Her husband fell in love with her all over again and wrote the doctor thank you letters once a year for saving her life and saving the marriage.

I loved the stories, but that day, tears were falling down my face because everything hurt, especially the pinching PICC-line in my arm and my stomach, which I was sure meant I now had stomach cancer. I could barely keep my head up, and I was about to undergo another three hours of poison dripping into my veins.

"Are you seeing someone?" the doctor asked kindly. This was New-York-speak for a shrink, someone who could help me through all this sadness, all these feelings. It was what we did in this part of New York with an excess of emotion. I had been doing it on and off all my life.

I nodded and wiped my soggy face.

The Poor Shrink

Every six weeks since the troubles started I had been seeing a psychiatrist to get antidepressants, and my insurance reimbursed me for almost all of his 450-dollar fee. He was a kind, bright, competent young doctor, referred by a friend who had been his supervisor. He was helpful in early stages preparing for the hospital, but once that was done, it was difficult to connect with him in talk therapy without irony. I was too aware that I was old enough to be his mother and had spent more years talking to shrinks than he had been alive.

When I described my reluctance to have visitors or contact friends whom I hadn't yet told I was sick, he said, "The problem is that your isolation is making this more difficult for you."

"I want something else to talk about, but it's the only thing I think about. I just want to fast forward through this and see them when it's over. If it's ever over." Poor me.

Poor shrink. I was cranky and inflexible with him, and I had done all the introspecting there was to do. My diagnosis was indisputable: I had cancer, a fucked-up gene, and the chemo blues, all of which meant I might die soon. And die at a much younger age than both my parents, who had smoked cigarettes for most of their lives. Plus, my stove didn't work.

When I went into the shrink's office and he'd ask, "How are you doing?" I'd answer, "Not so hot, how are *you*?"

It's embarrassing to think about how I acted out with him, but he was the only person getting paid, and paid handsomely, to listen to me, and why not express some of the anger and feelings of helplessness underneath my terror, which I usually tried to keep under wraps? And if I'd had to pinpoint the source of my anger, it was that I had gone so far as to use *organic* dental floss—and got cancer anyway. I'd gone to the trouble of being a lifelong hypochondriac and still got cancer. I knew all of this was utterly irrational, which was why I took such pains to keep it to myself most of the time. It was probably why I didn't want anyone to visit. But in the high-paid shrink's office—why not? He was used to dealing with people much more mentally unfit than I was. Still, I am not sure that expressing my anger to him did me much good. But he was right to schedule the appointments with me—I could have been doing much worse—and right to say the things he said. It wasn't his fault that, when I wasn't engrossed in a tawdry HBO miniseries or terrified that my stomach ache was stomach cancer, I was mad at the universe.

"Yes," I said now to the kindly chemo doctor, "I'm seeing someone, but it's just crying now, nothing serious. Aren't I too weak for a treatment today? Are you sure my body can take this?"

"You're fine," he said. "You just have to push through. Just one more treatment after today. You'll be ninety percent yourself three months from now."

Later, in the tiny exam room with the nurse, I mentioned that the PICC-line, the catheter drooping off my arm like a dead tulip, had pinched for two solid months. "I hate these things," she said. "*Hate* 'em. Let's see if we can get rid of it." She examined my hand, tapping on the veins. "Those look good. Very good. Let's see if we can get the IV going here, and then I'll take out the PICC."

While she went about the process of extracting the assortment of equipment that had been lodged into my veins of my upper arm and that made bathing a gymnastic event, I kept my eyes closed and gritted my teeth against the pain.

"Keep breathing," she said, "until I tell you to hold your breath."

It was bliss. A bone corset coming off. An airplane landing after a turbulent flight.

It will make you humble, Deena had said, and you will learn something.

When I got home that night from the doctor's office and looked at the new Visa card that had come in the mail, my mouth went dry. I learned that the card would expire in November 2020, three years later. The numbers made me dizzy—11/2020. Which of us would last longer: the credit card or me?

Postcard #2

An awful thought: There's something I've come to like about this misery.

Up early this morning, as usual, famished (the steroids?), weighing 118 pounds, with the pointy hipbones of a runway model. Two slices of toast with butter I ate standing at the kitchen counter and still hungry. Staring at the cabinet, staring at nothing, an awful thought: I don't actually mind being as miserable as I am. No obligations. No one to look after. Nothing to plan. I don't have to answer emails. Sleep, eat, take all the pills at the right times, and stagger out and walk a few blocks for exercise. Life stripped down to essentials. When I think of

Deena doing this with a young child and a business to run, and all the women with children, the women alone, women with menial jobs, with no support and no money going through this hell, I am engulfed in gratitude.

Where Is My Husband?

"You're going to be fine," he says.

"Maybe."

"You are."

"But the shitty gene."

"It's stage one. And you have the best doctor in the world. He'll figure something out."

"But . . . are you worried?"

"No."

"Even a little?"

"I'm concerned, but I'm not afraid. I don't go there unless I have to. Everything we know is that you're going to be fine, even if you're not right now."

He did not waver in his belief or in the expression of his belief, yet he was not impatient with me about my own fears. He left the apartment almost every weekday morning to take classes or teach classes in a university program for retired people and often had lunch with friends in the program. He teaches two new courses every semester, preparing each class for months, and preparing each session with fiendish energy. He's a popular teacher, often getting fulsome letters of appreciation from people in his classes. Before I got sick, I was happy for him having this school and these people in his life—and many of them in my life—and I was happy for him once I got sick because I was too weak to go anywhere and not great company at home.

He was so insistent I was going to be fine that, when my troubles began, I asked him not to tell people in the program, except for one close friend. I didn't want him to be an object of sorrow. I didn't want people in his classes to try to read the fear they imagined was behind his organized, professorial exterior. Maybe they would be surprised or puzzled to know that he didn't have any fear, which seemed to me a bit far-fetched, but he professed to having none. On the other hand, he is the King of Calm. It is not a pose. He was not going to indulge in fear unless he had to, unless the facts screamed "disaster."

One day in late November, I ran into a woman in his program in a cramped drugstore on Broadway, where we ended up practically nose to nose. James and I had had a few meals with her and her husband, and she noticed me easily, even though my thick wool hat covered my head, forehead, and neck.

"How are you?" she said.

"Oh, just fine," I said. I was not trying hard for sarcasm, but she must have heard a twinge in my voice.

"Are you kidding?" she asked.

I floundered.

"I know you've been having a hard time," she said.

"How do you know?"

"James told us."

I was so startled to hear this that I have no recollection of what else I said to her, though I'm sure I got away as soon as I could. I was not upset that he told people when I had asked him not to. To the contrary, I was touched. I was stunned. It was as surprising as anything that had happened since the ordeal. He had a secret life. A secret life of needing people to know that he was . . . a man whose wife had can-cer. A man who needed to be handled with care.

A Piece of My Heart

The stomachache-I-was-sure-was-cancer that I had for two months went away in three days after a GI doctor told me to stop eating wheat and dairy. This left only three things to eat, two of which needed a stove to prepare, but I was so relieved and felt so much better, I didn't care. If I whisked a few eggs in a bowl and put it in the microwave, it turned into a puffy egg soufflé that was fun to eat and didn't make me sick—and reminded me that *I didn't have another cancer.* One was quite enough.

When I arrived at the doctor's office for the next—and final—treat-ment on December fourteenth, I didn't stagger and didn't need a wheelchair to get from the waiting room to the exam room. And when the three hours were up and I was filled with steroids and joy that the treatments were over, I hit the sidewalk and walked west in the cold. I had a few strands of hair underneath my winter hat and more energy than I'd had in months. Two blocks west of the doctor's office, I was steps from what had been for sixty years the Lenox School for Girls, which was now, according to a bronze plaque, The New York School for Interior Design. I stopped and studied the elegant stone entranceway. The deep red front doors to the stately building that were there in 1972 had been replaced by leaded glass panes embed-ded in heavy stained wood.

A piece of my heart is embedded somewhere inside those doors. Could I go in and ask to poke around and revisit the sight of so many dulcet memories? Would I even recognize what must have been done to the interior? I was giddy with joy at the fact that I was walking away from the treatments for the last time, and slightly teary, thinking about Sue Briskman and my long-gone parents and their long-gone troubles. My veins were shot through with a poisonous wonder drug called R-CHOP (which stands for rituximab, cyclophosphamide, hydroxydaunorubicin, Oncovin, and prednisone), which was slamming every cell in my body for the last time and would give me enough energy today to venture across Central Park in the middle of December. Today was not the day to request a tour of my former high school.

At four o'clock, the park's trees were bare, the Great Lawn was shades of brown and palest yellow, but the skyline looking south was crisp and bright and wondrous against a deepening blue sky on what would soon be the shortest day of the year. And there I was—*there I was!*—walking miles in the cold without difficulty, pumped up with prednisone, grace, and another force that was even more elemental and random. I had not been born rich or beautiful or to parents whose lives would be comfortable or kind, but in the closing days of that year, I might as well have been able to grab my dumb good luck in my hands.

When I got home a short time later, there was news from many quarters: a good number of the students I had worked with during the summer and fall had been admitted "early decision" into the colleges where they most wanted to go, including a few Ivies. I hadn't disappointed them. I hadn't freaked anyone out with Cancer Alerts. I hadn't fucked up my part of the deal. And according to Google Maps, the journey I had just taken on foot was "48 minutes, 2.3 mi" and "Mostly Flat." It had been thirty degrees out, clear blue skies with eight mile an hour winds. Someone in my family had been sick and was now getting better.

Cured, Sort of

Two weeks after the last treatment, on the last workday of 2017, a Friday, I had a follow-up appointment with the doctor, the medical superstar, the kibitzer, the sweetheart, the man who suggested I write a book about people who are left-handed.

"I would consider you cured," he said, "except for the gene. To be on the safe side, I want you to have a tiny little spritz of radiation."

Deena would have asked him what exactly he meant. She would have pinned him down. What should I do to keep it at bay? How soon might it return? If it returned, would it be the same kind of lymphoma? Would I have the same treatment? And while we're at it, what's the real story with this cockeyed gene? What do those thousand doctors know that I need to know?

I had a sense that the answers would all be shrugs, a long train of *I don't knows* and *It depends* because if he knew something more, he would tell me. The problem—the doctor had explained it many times—was that there was simply no data on treating someone with this wonky gene of mine. It was all *maybe this* but then again *maybe that*. And *Let's see what my thousand colleagues will say*. Two months before, when I'd told my sometime-psychiatrist about the gene, he'd asked its name.

"I'm not going to tell you," I said, without an ounce of snark or hostility. It was just a declarative statement.

His impassive face twitched in astonishment. "Why not? I can find out about it for you. I used to work in cancer research."

"I don't want to know more than I know. It 'spooks' the leading doctor in the field. That's more than enough for me. There's no data on whether the treatment is going to work. It's nothing personal. I told my husband he couldn't look up the gene on the Internet either."

The seduction of knowledge in the age of information—was that where the shrink was coming from? There was a dearth of information in the mid-1970s when Sontag was diagnosed with breast cancer, and in the mid-1980s when Deena was. They both did mountains of research and went far and wide for treatments, willing to experiment with their one and only lives because the options conventional medicine offered were so grim, and the warlike metaphors followed suit. Even in the mid-1980s, Sontag reports, doctors in Italy and France did not tell many patients that they had cancer, though that practice was ending in the US. Now it's gone because so many life-extending treatments are available for many cancers, and information of every kind is a click away. The appetite for information is profound, now that it is not 1930 or even 1978, and some of the news is excellent, and not all the metaphors are about battles and wars.

Maybe the difference between the shrink and me was generational: if information exists, he wants to know what it is. Or maybe it was more basic: I'm a hypochondriac, and he's a medical doctor who works in a hospital. Information about illnesses, even the worst of them, doesn't make him want to cover his ears and hide under his desk.

Deena

A few days into the new year, I saw on Facebook that a woman I knew slightly as a teenager and briefly in college had been diagnosed with acute myeloid leukemia and was hospitalized. Should I get in touch with her as a fellow patient who had just been through this? Would that be a comfort to either of us? My first instinct was to connect. But say what? "Me too"? Or "Me too, but not so bad"? This was exactly why I had avoided cancer support groups, why I had made Nora Ephron and Susan Sontag—their silence and their writing—my support group. How could I not compare my fate to live people in the room with me? How could I avoid the inevitability of jealousy or guilt or just the constant pressure of so many houses in flames? It preyed on me, whether to write to the woman from college.

A month later, while taking yoga classes to rebuild my strength and jellied muscles, another decision was easy. One day after class the teacher came over to my place as I rolled up my mat, his expression somber. He happened to be Deena's son, who owns a yoga studio in our neighborhood.

"Have you talked to my mother?" I shook my head. "Lung cancer. They're not even staging it." I sank back down to the floor.

The world invades our bodies, our lungs. Deena, whose office on 9/11 was across from the World Trade Center, had been on her way to work that day. That was her subway stop. Her office building was not destroyed, and she was permitted to make several trips there to gather files and papers. Months later, when the premises were deemed "cleaned and cleared," she returned to her office. Sometime later, I remember sitting at her dining room table, listening to the wheeze she had developed. Talking about the wheeze. "Listen," she said to me, took a breath, let it in, and let it out. We figured it had something to do with the pit downtown and the air she'd been breathing for months, but what could she do? I can hear the strange sound to this day.

Or maybe it wasn't the toxic air from the burning buildings that gave her the wheeze that turned into lung cancer. Maybe it was something else. She was almost eighty years old. She was a forty-year survivor of breast cancer. Cancer happens, and the older you are, the more it happens. The body gives way. Genes mutate. Things fall apart. But the air down there—she had inhaled plenty of it, and it might as well have been a Monsanto factory in West Virginia. I called her as soon as I got home. "I've been taking yoga at Stephan's studio to get my strength back," I began, "and he just told me."

OK, Deena, you were right. I'm learning something. I'm learning that the cancer baton goes back and forth, when it doesn't go round and round.

Postcard #3

Amit's been calling more often than usual to find out how I am, and now I'm happy to answer that question. Yesterday, he said he was going to India for several months and would stop in Vietnam to see Bradley on his way back. The words were barely out of his mouth before I said, "Can I meet you there?"

I invited myself—just like that—into their visit and their friendship, which is ten years older than Amit's and mine, which is forty years old. Bradley was Amit's high school English teacher in London.

Amit said, "Sure!" almost as quickly.

Will our respective spouses mind that we are considering meeting seven thousand miles away? And will Amit and Bradley feel intruded upon?

"I've wanted to go there forever," I said, "and it would be wonderful to be there with you and Bradley." These two English expats who had left England many decades before, Amit for the US and Bradley for Asia, were like brothers.

I had the best excuse in the world for my brazenness—and the worst. No need for any of us to say it aloud, including our spouses: this is Liz's cancer bonus, her chance to do something ballsy because she might not get the chance to do it again, now that cancer has made an appearance, because who knows when it might return for an encore?

Vietnam, Finally

I had been wanting to visit Vietnam since it first opened up to tourists in the early 1990s because I wanted to see it before it turned into Hong Kong, or its own version of skyscraper hell. I wanted to go again in 1995, when my first husband and I were going to adopt a child from there, but by then I was more interested in the child than the country. A year later when the marriage ended—a nice way of saying "when I left"—it pained me for years to think about going to Vietnam. All I could imagine was anticipatory grief at the sight of every child I would see. Each one was the child who wasn't mine. But once James and Emily moved into my life, and I grew closer to Emily, the sting of the missing child faded. In its place was my longtime curiosity about the country that James had no interest in visiting. The university tours I came across were too expensive, and I didn't have the nerve to go alone.

Amit had known my first husband, known him well, and had known about the child we did not adopt, but knew nothing about my feelings around visiting Vietnam. When he called that day to check on me because I'd been sick for six months, and casually mentioned his plan to see Bradley on his way home from India, he had no idea that I would leap at the chance, like a dog leaping to catch a fly in his mouth. The wonder was that I caught it.

Ground Glass?

Room B-130. Radiation Oncology. Instead of windows and natural light in the basement, there's a TV in the spacious waiting room that is always tuned to CNN; there are dressing rooms with lockers, treatment rooms with millions of dollars of state-of-the-art equipment that can see inside your body, like the crazy promise of X-ray glasses that used to be advertised on the backs of cereal boxes. The machine assigned to me looks like a gigantic KitchenAid mixer minus the beater blades. I lie underneath the overhang as it shoots beams of radiation into an area smaller than an egg yolk while technicians control it from another room, on the other side of the door that's a foot thick. On the ceiling are colorful decorations, a sort of light show for patients on their backs, and there's even a sound system.

The technicians had said, "Bring any CD you like, and we'll play it when you're here." I brought Bob Dylan's *Time Out of Mind*, and even though they usually forgot to put it on, I didn't care. I had heard the CD a hundred times, and these sweet young people had more important things to do: position me on the table, set up the equipment, and close the giant door behind them before the zapping began. It was more serious but less stressful than, say, going to the dentist. Just a matter of lying there for a few minutes with this space-age machine rotating, buzzing, and whirling around making strange noises, in search of that spot in the right axilla where the lymph nodes had gone all cancery on me.

During those seventeen mornings doing time in B-130, there were two notable events.

One morning in the waiting room, I thought I saw a man I'd been involved with in my twenties, and I froze. His distinctive head of tight black curls. The delicate hands that held the newspaper he was reading. What would I say or do if that was him sitting six feet from me, head down reading? When he looked up, I saw I was mistaken—the man I knew would be much older than this one—but that idea stuck with me: old lovers meet again in Radiation Onc. A rom-com for seniors. The possibilities for their past were endless, and several involved her once-luxurious head of hair.

The other notable event was my second conversation with my radiologist, after he asked me to take a seat beside his desk. "I was re-reading the report from the PET scan you had last month, and there are a few very minor issues I didn't notice when I first saw it. No signs of lymphoma, but there are a few small nodules in your lungs—probably nothing."

He showed me the few lines of text in the section called CHEST: "0.7 cm right upper lobe ground-glass nodule (image 82), without associated FDG uptake." Also: "Tree-in-bud opacities are seen in the anterior portion of the right middle lobe, with associated FDG avidity, max SUV 4.6."

"Ground glass?" I asked. How could that be a medical term?

"It refers to the opacity of the nodule. It's hazy rather than solid."

"Which means?"

"It could be inflammation. It could be scar tissue. But just to be on the safe side, here's a list of pulmonologists we recommend."

"Were these nodules on the last PET scan?"

He searched my electronic file and did not find the September scan the oncologist had ordered when I was first diagnosed—a reminder that my legendary doctor keeps his patient records in manila files, not computers, and therefore unavailable to the rest of the hospital without advance planning and a working fax machine.

"Do I need to see the pulmonologist right away?"

"No. These are very small nodules. He'd want you to do another scan, and you can't do one for a few months."

A joyous delay—even if the pulmonologist says these are not nothing, I'd be spared learning about them until after my upcoming trips. In mid-March, two weeks in Italy, then two weeks in Asia. I wasn't ready for another body melodrama, but I was sort of getting used to the ways of doctors—the enterprise they are engaged in. I mean, how they manage to work with such sick people without feeling crushed by the end of every day.

They read bodies, scans, and reports the way I read students' college essays, asking myself: "What are the problems here? How do we fix them?" Students show me their essays and wait, holding their breath, for my judgment, as though I am the admissions officer about to rule on their application. The doctors, solving problems in 3D, flip through reports looking for "issues" and "problems" to be addressed, as I flip through essays, neither of us in a position to grant the big prize—a clean bill of health, admission—but only to detect whatever imperfections might be marring the pictures before setting out to fix them. To the doctor and the essay coach, the document is a question mark, a problem that might need solving. To the patient and the college applicant, the document is life or death.

Actually, make it a third notable event. On day fourteen, one of the regular young technicians who walked me from the waiting room—where my ex-lover did not wait—to the treatment room stood at that door with his arm theatrically outstretched like a maître d' and said, "Table for one."

I smiled. I might even have laughed a little because it was the first jokey thing he'd said, after two weeks of daily encounters. "That's good," I said. "That's very funny."

I wish I'd asked him for more radiation treatment jokes. I bet there are a bunch of them, but I was never in my Girl Reporter mode at those times. I was slightly withdrawn, eager to do what they said, and did not feel at all bouncy or talkative. I didn't want to distract them while they arranged my body to get the beams landing in the right place. And everywhere I went, from the waiting room to the dressing room, past the technician's stations in my hospital gown, not to mention inside The Room with the Machine, I was that most unenviable of people, the Cancer Patient. It did not exactly put a spring in my step.

I was no longer as actively terrified as I had been six months before, but I was more than a little uneasy that my prognosis had a loophole in it big enough to drive a Subaru through. But to the extent I felt like I was *fighting a battle against cancer*, during the time I spent in Radiation Onc being zapped by a million-dollar machine, I knew I had military might on my side. I hoped it meant that maybe, just maybe, I would win, though I kept that thought, and most others, to myself.

Part
Three

Where Did It Go?

I first noticed a change as James and I prepared for a trip to Rome in March 2018, a few days after the treatments ended. It was strange. As I thought about the trip, as I packed, gathered tickets, notebooks, and gadgets, I felt nothing but excitement. It was as though, along with all the weight I had dropped, I lost the fear of flying. As the plane from JFK lifted off the ground, I did not start a nervous conversation with the stranger sitting next to me, as I often did, to calm my rattling nerves. As we touched down in Rome, I was not so overwrought that tears came to my eyes, having survived another near-death experience. Two weeks later, when we landed at JFK, it was a decidedly *Hey, no problem* landing. Which was not a small miracle but actually more of a large one. I would get to test my new shock absorbers a week later, when I flew on my own to Vietnam and, after five days with Amit and Bradley, test them again on a short flight to Cambodia, where I had long wanted to go the temples of Angkor Wat.

Where had it gone, all this fear? Had I only been allotted so much at birth, and after so many units of cancer fear, now it was mostly gone, like women eventually running out of ova that can be fertilized? Or had surviving cancer—moving through all that fear and coming out on the other side in a state of "cured, but"—made me a sturdier person, one with a new layer of calloused skin that was not easily punctured? Was I like someone who had gotten a black belt in judo and felt safer walking in dodgy neighborhoods, even though judo could not repel a bullet? Could the endorphins from feeling so powerful have flushed out my fears?

Postcard #4

We are staying in the oldest hotel in Vietnam, the Continental Saigon in Ho Chi Minh City, built in 1880 and never tarted up to look like the antiseptic twenty-first century. It sparkles with polished wood floors and bannisters, high ceilings, French windows, heavy wooden furniture that has an "Oriental" feel, and layered beige draperies that look like they're from the 1930s. Down the hall from me is Room 214, where Graham Greene wrote part of *The Quiet American* in 1951, says the plaque by the door. The hotel bar was a gathering place for reporters during the war in the 1960s, and a famous spy lived on the third floor. Breakfast is a lavish buffet of croissants, dragon fruit, pho, and the best coffee I've ever had.

Bradley, who is 80 years old and six feet tall, lives in a high rise in the suburbs and comes into the city, which he calls Saigon, on the back-of-a-motorcycle taxi service. The driver is always a foot shorter than he is—a balancing act for the two of them. We go to art galleries, museums, and restaurants, but these are merely settings for conversation, what Amit calls "walking pedagogy." Teacher and student have been talking literature and politics for fifty years, and when I'm with them, I'm certain I have stumbled into a Merchant-Ivory film on the banks of the Saigon River.

Gleaming with Survivorship

I came home on a high. Not only the adventure of the trip but the fact that, on my two flights back, my paralyzing fear was still nowhere to be found. In the wake of the trip, my thoughts went to the extreme of the chemotherapy as an explanation for this sudden absence: the body blow of the chemical drips, its unrelenting harshness, the exhaustion, the drama of crawling my way back, and how difficult it was to believe that I would ever recover from something so debilitating, so total. What it must be like to be in a crushing accident, every limb in traction, immobilized, and to imagine one day playing tennis. *It will never happen.* A few months earlier, I couldn't walk from 84th Street to 83rd Street, but I had just walked six miles a day in blistering pre-monsoon heat and humidity through Asia. My accomplishment, my mini-Mount Everest.

As I tried to make sense of my trip and of my state of mind, the theme of going to extremes set off a tripwire: Cancer. Chemotherapy. Vietnam. The Vietnam War had been the soundtrack of my youth, and the country was the home of the child I came so close to adopting more than twenty years earlier, a plan I quashed when I understood I had to leave my husband, that his moods and depression were contagious, that I could not raise a child with him. Leaving him was the hardest thing I had ever done, knowing I was his lifeline but knowing I would go down with him if I stayed. The husband whose cause of death was "inconclusive" but could have been suicide. The years I spent after he died, wondering what to do with the role of the "almost widow" that was mine, and out of which came my novel *Almost*. I had been more than a wide-eyed tourist exploring Ho Chi Minh City. I was visiting his distant past and a piece of my own. I was making my own history there. And when I saw children on the street, I did not grieve. The one who would have been mine was now thirty years old.

Going to these extremes might have blown my circuits, left my overworked amygdalae in tatters; maybe I was too wiped out to be afraid. Or was it the opposite? Was I emboldened by surviving the chemo, smacking down the cancer—Sontag called her mood after her first cancer "gleaming with survivorship"—so I had no more truck with that hoary fear of mine? Or had I come so close to the possibility of my own death that I figured my odds of dying from cancer were greater than the odds of dying in a plane crash?

Oh, the Places You Didn't Go

Years ago, my friend Evelyn and her husband were visiting the US, but ended up with different return flights back to England that were separated by a few hours. We'd gone out to JFK for drinks with them, and his plane left before hers. As he said goodbye to us, husband and wife kissed quickly and mumbled, "See you at Heathrow," and we visited a bit longer with Evelyn. The utterly banal moment was anything but for me. I could not have done it so casually—gotten on a separate plane from James as though it were a bus or a subway, and we'd soon meet up again at 59th Street. I would have said goodbye—not making a scene but torn up inside—as though I was boarding a transport train to Poland in 1943.

Despite my fear, I traveled many places—always convinced I wouldn't make it home. The last five or ten minutes of nearly every flight were intense. By that time, we were nearly on the ground, and I could believe *we would make it*. I could see the runway, knew the pilot was in control. In another minute or two, this vigilance, this anticipation of disaster, would be over. When the wheels kissed the ground, I was so wrung out, so relieved, that tears often came to my eyes, such was my gratitude after the certainty, spread out over the length of the trip, that I was going to my death. Every landing was a reprieve, the governor commuting my execution a minute before midnight.

Decades ago, at National Airport going to visit my grandparents in Hartford, I was so fearful that I didn't board the plane, didn't take the trip. And then there were the exotic travels I denied myself, including Thailand, when I was writing a novel that was set there, and Argentina, when a friend who was the US ambassador invited James and me to stay with her in the ambassador's residence. I had a hankering to see Chile, and after learning about Shackleton's expeditions and reading about poet Diane Ackerman's visit there, I yearned, like the character in *Where'd You Go, Bernadette?* for Antarctica. Given the extent of my fears, it was a wonder I went where I went, which included Hong Kong, Turkey, St. Petersburg, Scandinavia, and, dozens of times, England and Europe. But the places I *didn't go*—they told the story of someone much more adventurous, the story of my unlived lives.

Speaking of Fear

From Mel Brooks and Carl Reiner's *2000 Year Old Man*:

> MEL BROOKS. Everything we do is based on fear.
>
> CARL REINER: Even love?
>
> MB: Mainly love.
>
> CR: How can love stem from fear?
>
> MB: What do you need a woman for? You know what you need a woman for? In my time, to see if an animal is behind you. . . . You say to a lady, "Lady, would you look behind me for a while?" . . . "OK, how long you want?" "Forever. OK, we're married."
>
> CR: What was the means of transportation back then?
>
> MB: Fear . . . an animal would growl, and you would go two miles in a minute.

This Is What They Said When I Asked

The Boston Strangler, a panic attack, riding elevators and subways, Nazis coming down the street, my father's rage, my mother's empty eyes, dying alone, losing my intellectual acuity, a past indiscretion will come back to haunt me, not being talented enough, my children having to struggle, losing my "version" of any story, people being angry at me, aging because with it comes invisibility and all that entails, losing my memory, hurting people through my own failings, homelessness, I will get sick and my children will not take care of me or visit me, poverty, abandonment, being raped, being ax-murdered, never doing anything significant, death of a loved one.

These are some of the answers I received from ten women when I posted a question on my Facebook page: "What are the top 2–3 things you're most afraid of? Do they involve your health, your children, your finances? All 3? Is 3 far too few? Would you consider yourself a hypochondriac?"

Some were childhood fears, most were present-day. I was struck that no one answered "cancer," "debilitating illness," or "flying." I was struck at how ready people—women, including some I'd never communicated with before—were to share on Facebook and emails. I was not surprised that no one answered, "being killed by police" or "that my children would be killed by police," because, as far as I knew, the women who answered my question were white. And no one had answered, "being molested/raped by my boss/professor," because, from what I knew, the responders were mostly women who were either self-employed or retired. Some lists were very long and detailed, and one mentioned the aftereffects of having been raped.

In the hierarchy of emotions, fear is the among the most primitive. It's processed through the amygdalae, two almond-shaped clusters of nuclei deep in the temporal lobes of the cerebrum, right next to the hippocampus, which controls memory. Frightening events pulsing through the amygdalae seep into the hippocampus and take up residence in our memories. That's why I can remember flying into Denver years ago in a lightning storm, the plane bouncing through the sky, but I can no longer remember why I was going to Denver. Why I can remember the actual sensation of picking up the phone one afternoon in 1996, two months after my divorce was final, and the speaker announcing he was with the Massachusetts State Police, and I knew this meant my ex-husband was dead. When I understood the proximity of the amygdalae to the hippocampus, it made sense that frightening events become such clear memories and that prolonged or repeated painful incidents can cause intractable trauma.

The answers to my Facebook question reminded me of people who are fearless in patently dangerous situations—Sontag visiting Sarajevo eleven times during the Bosnian War, yet afraid to sleep in the dark when she had cancer. A friend fears her daughter is dead if she is more than ten minutes late and yet feels perfectly safe in airplanes. And those who are not afraid of public speaking (me) but are afraid of speaking privately to doctors (me). As I remember and record here how tongue-tied, how paralyzed, I was when talking to doctors, I wonder how differently my story might have gone if I had been a mini-Deena, pinning the doctors down, asking for specifics instead of clamming up. Or if I had just been the plucky, inquisitive person I am in every situation other than the one I was in, when I was literally scared to death.

REWRITING ILLNESS | 163

The Literature of Fear

In the vast literature of fear—which includes academic studies, reruns of *The Dick Van Dyke Show*, and the observations of my grandmother—we learn that men and women are typically afraid of different things and express their fears differently. In an unfunny moment, comedian Amy Schumer says that women are afraid of being attacked, and men of being ridiculed. When women fear men, they often fear they will be hurt physically. When men fear women, they brace for emotional pain. It's no secret that jealousy and imagined jealousy trigger violence in violent men. And we know from nearly every phone call with a woman friend that women often ruminate on fears to the point of perseverating, while men, faced with the same situation, predictably switch to "problem-solving mode"—and promptly fall asleep. I exaggerate, but not by much.

As much time as I've spent considering sex-linked fears, I never gave a moment's thought to doctor-linked fears until later in this journey, despite my own doctor being "spooked" by my wayward gene. Doctors don't go around wearing their fears on their sleeves the way patients do. For one thing, they know that we don't want our authority figures to tell us they're terrified. Or even spooked. They're the pilots, and if they're not sure how to fly the plane, we'd rather not know.

As easy as it was for me to be angry at some of my doctors for what they had done and hadn't done early in my illness, I did not see any of it through the lens of their training and their own fears until much later, when I read Atul Gawande's book, *Being Mortal: Medicine and What Matters in the End*, and specifically a passage early on:

The one time I remember discussing mortality was during an
hour we spent on *The Death of Ivan Ilyich*, Tolstoy's classic
novella. It was in a weekly seminar called Patient-Doctor—part
of the school's effort to make us more rounded and humane
physicians. Some weeks we would practice our physical
examination etiquette; other weeks we'd learn about the effects of
socioeconomics and race on health. And one afternoon we
contemplated the suffering of Ivan Ilyich as he lay ill and
worsening from some unnamed, untreatable disease.

This sentence fragment spooks me: "The one time I remember discussing mortality was during an hour we spent on . . ."

An hour, Dr. Gawande? Are you kidding me? Then it's no wonder
the psychiatrist responded as he did when I complained about the
doctors who blithely told me they didn't think I had cancer: "Liz, you
know that doctors have a hard time giving people bad news."

They are in the business of bad news—of illness itself—but receive
almost no training in how to talk to people about it, especially when
the end is near. The training, especially now with so many medical
advancements, is to keep people alive for as long as possible, often by
any means necessary, and often when a candid conversation about
what lies ahead would be wiser than another crushing round of chemo. But it's easier to suggest or agree to the chemo—"One more
try!"—and it takes less time and emotional energy than bringing up
The Talk No One Wants to Have. Dr. Gawande recalls a patient near
death whose sister asked if the woman was dying:

I didn't know how to answer the question. I wasn't even sure
what the word "dying" meant anymore. In the past few decades,
medical science has rendered obsolete centuries of experience,

tradition, and language about our mortality and created a new difficulty for mankind: how to die.

In the course of the book, with guidance from someone skilled in such discussions, Dr. Gawande learns to get past his fears and think differently about what matters at the end of life. And he learns—much to his astonishment—that letting death take its course without endless interventions can extend life and improve the process of dying for patients and loved ones. People hooked up to machines or being flattened by chemo in order to cadge extra time often have less time—and less quality time—than those who spend their last weeks or months connecting in meaningful ways with loved ones.

It was my great good fortune that no doctor had to tell me I had a terminal illness, but the skittishness of many physicians and what felt to me at times like being gaslighted—though I know no malevolence was involved—made much more sense once I understood the limitations of their training and the philosophy behind it. Medical instruction is about saving lives; any life is better than death—and treatments are easier to discuss than Letting Go. In fact, I was incredibly touched to read about how difficult these conversations were for Dr. Gawande. Touched to read about how hard he tried to learn a new way of relating to patients—including, eventually, his dying father. And touched to know that my doctors—who seemed for such a long time to hold all the cards and have all the answers—had something in common with me: their silence too came from fear. Which meant that The 2000 Year Old Man was right again: *Everything we do is based on fear.*

Whether it's doctors' distinct fears or women's or my own, I sometimes think that if fear could be converted into an energy source like coal or gas, it could power the planet—or maybe it already does.

Hmmmm

"Did you have TB as a child?" the pulmonologist wanted to know, studying the new June 2018 scan of my lungs with their ground glass nodules and a large blob next to them that he thought was inflammation. He moved his bifocals slowly up and down as he tried to make sense of the shadings and shapes he saw in the multiplicity of views on the screen, which made as much sense to me, looking over his shoulder, as a Rorschach test.

"No," I answered.

"Are you sure?"

"Very sure. Just ordinary things like mumps."

Eyes squinting, he emitted a "Hmmmm," which did not fill me with confidence, then said, "Well." Another bold pronouncement. "As I said, this larger shape could be inflammation." He pointed to the smaller smudges, the ground glass. "These nodules over here could be scar tissue or inflammation or low-grade lung cancer."

Nice that he mentioned cancer at the end of the list. But you wouldn't say, "It could be cancer or it could be a blister." You'd always mention the blister first, saving the tough stuff for later in the sentence. And there was the comforting adjective "low-grade," which meant I could dissolve into a low-grade, slo-mo panic rather than a full-blown cancer meltdown.

But I said nothing and thought of Deena, who would ask a dozen questions, and who was whispering in my ear to ask something, ask anything. *Speak up!* she said in a stage whisper, although she was nowhere to be seen. But my fear made me mute—that, and I knew that I'd be scanned in another six months, and the scans are where the truth lies. Everything else I might discuss with the doctor now was chatter, unless I wanted a lesson on low-grade cancers and how they grow—which I did not. I was plenty spooked enough.

"There's nothing to worry about now," the pulmonologist said, "but make sure to send me any scans you have."

As I walked up York Avenue, past the many edifices of Weill Cornell, where I knew Deena was being treated for cancer so advanced it was beyond staging, I imagined her peppering the doctors with questions. Were they her version of nervous chatter in the face of a terrible diagnosis, as though nestled into one of those comments might be a ray of hope? I could talk to her about almost anything—but not that, not now. I had to return to these mean streets the next morning for my six-month follow-up, and I would have to report the "low-grade lung cancer" possibility so the doctor could add it to my hefty manila file.

Eighteen Months to Go

There was never a day I didn't worry. Never two days in a row when I didn't cross my hands over my chest and slide my hands snugly into my armpits to catch anything sprouting there in its early stages. I'd be sure to outsmart it this time, catch the next lump long before it grew to golf ball-size. Armpits clear, I'd brush the skin at the top of my inner thighs, where lymph nodes flourish. Did I have a fever? Why did my forehead itch? And my calf? Was my back ache just a pulled muscle or did I have lymphoma in my bones? When I saw TV commercials about cancer centers and cancer drugs, I'd turn the sound off and look away. But there was one I had memorized. One man's lymphoma did not respond to chemo and had to be treated with a transplant. But that wasn't me—my lumps had gone away, though they might come back. Any day. And if they did, would I need a transplant—on 10 South—or just more chemo—on 10 North? And if I had to take more chemo, would its toxicity cause another cancer, which doctors believed was the reason for the appearance of Susan Sontag's second cancer a decade after her first, or was it her third?

When fear of cancer was merely a hypochondriac's closest friend, I didn't know that the disease—speaking of metaphors—was like the coast of Maine, a landscape so full of intricacies and hidden coves, crevices, and dangers, that it can never be accurately measured or fully known. Yet once I'd come down with it and gotten through it, I mostly managed to keep the most pressing of its terrors at bay, though I had fleeting out-of-body reminders: I shuddered when I saw the dates my passport and credit cards were going to expire. Would I beat them to the finish line?

My visit the next day was with Dr. D., my new official doctor. He had looked after me briefly the year before when his partner was out of town. Though they worked in the same office, their finances were different. Dr. D. was in my insurance network, which meant one less pressure point on my nervous system.

"The bloodwork is fine, and the PET scan looks great," Dr. D. said, after ten or fifteen minutes of schmoozing about my summer plans and his. He is a big-hearted man who seems to have time on his hands, though the office waiting room is usually packed with patients divided up between several doctors. I knew he meant that the PET scan looked great vis-à-vis my lymph system.

"Except for the ground glass nodules in my lungs," I said.

"So we'll keep an eye on those."

"Are you sure there's nothing else in the PET scan to worry about?" It was fun talking to a doctor about my summer plans, but I was afraid that he might be distracted by them and miss something.

His eyes scanned the page again. "I don't see anything that concerns me. And if you make it through the first two years without a recurrence, there's a good chance it won't come back."

"Even with my terrible gene?" I asked.

He nodded. "There are ways to abrogate it."

I couldn't quite believe what I was hearing and wondered when this had happened, this incredible news about the gene no longer being a menace to me. Would I have to take a pill, get an operation, have a microchip implanted? True to form, I didn't ask him to elaborate because I was afraid that any answer might have a piece of upsetting information tucked into it. Or was it because I didn't quite believe him? If something so dramatic had happened—my spooky, life-threatening gene was no longer a problem?—why hadn't they told me? Or maybe he just had? I think I said, "Wow." Or maybe I didn't. Maybe I just thought it. Or maybe I was flooded with information and emotion and couldn't think clearly. Plus, the doctor had delivered the news so off-handedly. Oh, by the way, that gene that spooked the hell out of the other doctor—*no problem!*

Wow. But still, eighteen more months. Eighteen months in which to keep holding my breath.

"It's a good time to be alive!" exclaimed Dr. D.

I did not spread this news widely. No texts, no emails, no pretty botanical postcards. There were still miles to go, and I didn't want to get my hopes up only to have them crushed if the disease returned.

Didn't want friends to have this date hovering over their thoughts about me. I had enough of my own anxiety looking at the calendar and checking off the months.

A good time to be alive?

I'll let you know.

Celebrity Sighting

One excellent spring afternoon, I met a writer friend visiting from the West Coast for lunch at Boulud Sud near Lincoln Center. We were not intimates but she'd contributed an essay to one of my anthologies, *What My Mother Gave Me*. In our several meals together, we had talked for hours.

"So what've you been up to?" she said, glancing from the menu to the tony surroundings.

Not usually a trick question, though it was that day.

I had not planned my answer, but it was almost like flipping an internal coin, deciding which way to go. I'd worn the wig I rarely wore rather than a cancer hat, which would have led to questions, so I was already leaning toward *skip the cancer*. But was there something about friendship and intimacy that demanded the truth?

"The usual reading and writing," I said, my mind made up, "and trips to Italy and Vietnam."

Stories fell off our tongues as we talked about books and editors and writers, between bites of fattoush and chicken tagine and pretending we were ladies who lunch instead of writers who usually eat yogurt at our computers. And I knew that if I said one word—and it happened to be *cancer*—the entire lovely lunch would take a nose-dive. It would become My Cancer Story. When we talked briefly about *Me, My Hair and I,* my friend gazed at my hair and said, "You're rocking the gray hair," and I bit my tongue not to tell her it was a wig because, well, by the way, I had cancer. There was my moment to ruin the meal, but I resisted, and moments later, I spotted Natalie Portman and her family a few tables away from us. "Look, look who's there!" We were giddily starstruck when Natalie's toddler scampered past our table, one of her grandparents hard at her heels, while Natalie zipped ahead to the restaurant's entrance. For ten minutes, we watched their every move.

If you are in the business of creating and crafting scenes—in novels, memoirs, even college essays—this was one I much preferred to the cancer-confession-over-the-hummus vignette. For one thing, I did not have to explain that my prognosis at the moment was *Cured but.* Or that I had seventeen or eighteen months left in which to learn whether the darn thing was likely to come back again. The less said about the big C, the more fun it was for me. And for my friend, though she didn't know it. Nora Ephron's resounding silence kept making sense.

"What If You Die When I'm at School?"

Limbo bore a striking resemblance to ordinary life, made easier because only three or four people knew anything about my lousy gene, the ticking clock, the mental calendar whose months I ticked off as they ended, and no one was paying as close attention as I was. December 2018: another six-month exam with Dr. D., which I was sure would be followed by a PET scan. The protocol was that in the first two years following treatment, scans are every six months.

"That's changed," Dr. D. told me during the exam. "The new research says that as long the bloodwork and the physical are fine—and there are no other symptoms—a PET scan isn't necessary every six months." The news was a stunning relief. Not having to take a PET scan is almost as thrilling as getting a clean one. That day, I passed the physical and the multiple-choice checklist: no swellings, no night sweats, no itching or weight loss. I was elated—but told only James. Math is math: twelve months down and twelve to go.

A few weeks after seeing the doctor, my gleaming-with-survivorship endorphins were still strong enough to get me onto flights to Miami and then Israel, without feeling the old certainty that I was going to my execution. In Israel, I would see my parents' oldest friend, who had recently moved from Hartford to Jerusalem to be near her expat daughter, and I would meet dozens of cousins in the country of my paternal grandfather's birth. He had been born there in 1899 when it was Palestine, under Ottoman rule. He and his siblings left several years later for the US, but one sibling returned in 1932 and married into another Jewish family. She had two sons whose children and grandchildren I had never met but who were close to many of our relatives in Hartford. As a nonobservant Jew who had married not one but two non-Jewish men, I had long been reluctant to visit. I was afraid I would not feel comfortable with my relatives in their country. Now, having visited Vietnam and Cambodia, and having survived my illness, at least for now, it lingered as A Place I Need to Go. Never mind my failing grades in Judaism.

It was—but how could it not be?—an exhilarating, illuminating trip. Our relatives gathered every cousin for a potluck Shabbat dinner the night after we arrived in Tel Aviv. The table was laden with salads, pastas, gigantic strawberries, and a dozen pints of Ben and Jerry's ice cream. Someone had found a way to translate "Chunky Monkey" into Hebrew. There were no tests, no quizzes, no religious hoops to jump through. I was Uncle Sam's granddaughter. Nothing else mattered.

James and I were ardent tourists, staying in hotels in Tel Aviv and Jerusalem, visiting museums and religious sights, and even hiring several private guides, including one who showed us around Bethlehem on the West Bank. I did not mention my illness to anyone there. Nor did I mention what I was writing—what became this memoir. When people asked what I was working on, I mentioned that the editor of *Salmagundi* had asked me to write an essay about the upcoming twentieth anniversary of Bill Clinton's impeachment—reflections on what it meant then and now. It was easier to dwell on Bill and Monica through the ages than to bring cancer into the conversation. What I lacked in candor, I made up for being cheerful company, keeping the focus off my troubles. I was not exactly rewriting my history, just editing it for the occasion.

Within days of returning, I heard from Deena's son, Stephan, about her condition. She had spent the last year in every kind of treatment, seizing every last moment of joy she could, the most spectacular of which was Bill T. Jones' marathon dance, *Analogy Trilogy*, where she sat in the audience ecstatically watching from her wheelchair for seven hours. By the end of January 2019, she was confined to a reclining chair in her bedroom overlooking Riverside Park.

"She's pretty close to the end," Stephan told me.

He and his wife, Ingrid, had a part-time hospice nurse, but they were her primary caregivers. They lived on the other side of the apartment in a large bedroom with their daughter, in the space where I had lived part-time for many years, renting the room, becoming family-close to Deena. "We're arranging visits from people who want to say goodbye to her. We've got about forty people so far. I know she wants to see you."

She was almost eighty and had so many people to say goodbye to because she'd had a big, bold, purpose-filled life. Back when the Upper West Side was more like Charles Bronson's *Death Wish* than Nora Ephron's *You've Got Mail*, she owned a neighborhood pottery studio with hundreds of students and artists. Later on, she had a radio show on WBAI about New York politics while working a full-time job in which she had organized a network of public schools and community organizations to feed 250,000 New York City kids school lunches and summer meals. All of that was before her fourth or fifth career as a life coach. When Stephan was growing up, she and a group of young New York families rented a big house on Shelter Island every summer for fifteen years, and she was still connected to some of the parents and the adult children. Not to mention the women whose names and talents were described in the huge, well-thumbed loose-leaf binder on her desk: a vast network of women willing to barter everything from house cleaning and jewelry-making to legal help.

Months before the end, she filed claims with two organizations that awarded money to people who had become sick from living or working near the demolished World Trade Center. In her last month, she was overwhelmed with paperwork for her claims. By the time I saw her, she had a hard time using even a phone, but she was alert, articulate, and unafraid to talk about her state of mind, her imminent death, and her seven-year-old granddaughter, who, with her parents, had been reading an assortment of children's books about dying.

"We've been talking about this for months," Deena said calmly. "The other day, she said to me, 'Grandee, what will happen if you die when I'm at school?' I said, 'It'll be just fine, sweetheart, because I'll be with you. I'll *always* be with you.' When I told her that, she was fine."

After a long pause, Deena said, "I have been *so* lucky. So *so* lucky." Though in so many ways, she hadn't been. Divorced with a young child. Constant money troubles. And decades before, the love of her life had died of a heart attack. "To live with a child again. To see the world through her eyes as she tries to make sense of everything. What a joy. What an incredible gift it's been."

And I had been so lucky to live in that room from the time right after my divorce in 1996 through many years into my relationship with James, whom I met in 1999. In the early years, I lived there full-time and then less often as I began going to Boston to stay with James. In all those years, Deena's apartment and that bedroom, which she had always rented out, were the only home I had, as my divorced parents lived separately in one-bedroom apartments from the time I graduated from high school until they died. She and I were roommates, friends, confidants, and then, in a plot twist we couldn't have foreseen, cancer sisters.

Did Deena's fearlessness carry over into her dying? Yes, if fearlessness is the ability to confront death without denial. And though she and Sontag had a few fearless genes in common, their paths diverged sharply in Sontag's refusal to acknowledge that she was dying, even at the end. In his moving memoir, *Swimming in a Sea of Death*, her son, David Rieff, writes: "Almost until the moment she died, we talked of her survival, of her struggle with cancer, never about her dying. I was not going to raise the subject unless she did. It was her death, not mine. And she did not raise it."

Deena was hyper-conscious and verbal about what she was going through at every stage, no longer asking questions of the pilots, the experts, but charting her own journey to the last stop. After she died, Ingrid told me that in those last weeks, Deena put on a brightly colored blouse every morning until the day she chose a black one—which turned out to be the last blouse she put on. There was no denial in her departure.

Shortly after Deena died, Ingrid wrote a long, detailed Facebook post that moved me beyond measure. In a voice that matched Deena's in clarity and surpassed hers in emotional intensity, Ingrid described Deena's last days and final hours in her struggle to let go, a tug of war between Deena and Death. Ingrid recounted the ways she and Stephan, who had spent time working in a hospital cancer ward, nursed Deena through her excruciating departure, a pair of midwives engaged in a long, grueling unbirth. She had made her peace with dying, but she did not go gently.

The story and Ingrid's telling are a testament to Deena's power to live and die with more boldness than fear and inspire those around her to do the same, even if not all of us had her aplomb. Two weeks later, at the end of the service that Stephan and Ingrid held at their yoga studio, they handed out small red envelopes, the size of business cards, each with a pinch of Deena's remains. I put mine in a small pocket on the side of my purse, for the next time I was near an ocean. Where else should Deena be laid to rest?

Postcard #5

I keep the windows open even in February, hoping some of Deena's and Ingrid's passion will blow my way from two blocks south, hoping it will help me find a voice for the fourth draft of this story. I'm working from earlier drafts, plucking lines and paragraphs here and there. But I still don't know how the story might end, which will dictate the telling, the voice, the tone. It's true that no one gets out of here alive, but how soon do I have to face my departure? How many visits to 10 North or 10 South will end up on my dance card?

I take a yogurt from the fridge, sit down, stare at the screen, at the swirls of yogurt, at the spoon. Being in limbo is not a story. Waiting is not a story. At the moment, it's like building a house when you don't know the style or how many floors it will have. Like trying to hang a door before you know whether it will open in or out.

Fourteen months down, ten to go.

Clearing Things Up: Thing One: The Secret Lives of Doctors

One morning in April 2019, I returned to the towering Tisch Cancer Center at Mount Sinai—a hardened cancer veteran by now—to see the surgeon who did the biopsy of my lymph node almost two years before. I needed two things: his opinion about the parathyroid problem that had been eclipsed by the lymph node problem, and a clarification of a comment he made the year before.

Having an overactive parathyroid keeps the bones from absorbing calcium. For many people, the calcium floating around the bloodstream instead of seeping into the bones causes intense fatigue, but I had never had that symptom. I just had a mildly high calcium reading and a very high parathyroid hormone number. But after many years of this, I now had the beginnings of osteoporosis.

The surgery to fix this is frightening and involves removing one, two, or three of the four parathyroid glands, each the size of a lentil, that are located at the front of the throat. And the doctor will not know which glands to remove until he opens me up and tests each for its activity or hyperactivity. In my case, nothing definitive was evident from the scans, which showed only the faintest irregularity.

I was there to ask the surgeon if the procedure could wait eight more months, until my Medicare started in December 2019, when I could do it without expensive co-pays or hospital charges.

It was a relief to see him with cancer behind me, a lion loping in the other direction instead of staring right at me. He looked at my bone density scan and my blood work and declared, "It would be fine to wait until December."

One matter down, one to go. "Do you mind if I ask you a question?" I ventured.

"Ask away."

"When I first came here," I said calmly, "you wanted me to get a biopsy of the lump, and I asked if it could wait until after my vacation. You said it would be fine to wait, and that you didn't think I had cancer. Did you really not think I had cancer?"

"I don't remember saying that, but if you say so, then I did. I thought there was a chance you had cancer, but if I told you that you didn't, it was only so that you could enjoy your vacation a little more. *And because I knew you would come back here.* I wasn't worried that you'd drop this." A pause, a thoughtful pause. Another memory? "I have a patient now who keeps postponing a test he needs, and I had to say to him the other day, 'I think this is cancer, and if you don't do something about it now, you are *going to die.*' That was the only way I could get his attention. It worked."

Oh.

Oh.

Oh.

The secret lives of doctors.

He had me pegged after all, and I had him pegged.

Our exchange had an ending with a few twists. The doctor lied about my cancer so I could have a more carefree vacation, but instead all I did was wonder whether he'd been lying to me. At the same time, I was touched to hear that he had made a judgment about me that was correct; I would return to his office once I got home from the beach.

We don't get to rewrite the past, but based on what he had just told me, do I wish he had shaded his pre-vacation comment in the leaning-cancer rather than the I-don't-think-so direction? How much worse would I have felt leaving town for three weeks if he had said, "There's a chance you have cancer, but it won't make a difference if we don't find out until a month from now"? If he'd gone with *leaning-cancer*, I would not have wondered if he was lying to me, which might have resulted in more fear but less cognitive dissonance. I would have done fewer jumping jacks in the driveway of the cottage, hoping to shrink my swollen lymph nodes. I would have had a different conversation with Kate, my nurse practitioner friend. I would have obsessed instead over what *kind* of cancer I probably had, rather than whether the doctor was lying. For the doctor, I suppose the choice was easy, a throwaway: give her a few more weeks of uncertainty, maybe even of hope, before the truth comes crashing down.

We don't get to rewrite the past, only to wonder what might have been.

What *should* the doctor have said that day in his office as I was about to leave town?

Who's in charge of how doctors should talk to patients about cancer and about what *might* be cancer? It was simple back when patients were lied to because there was so little to do. Nowadays, truth prevails. But what about in the time between symptoms and diagnosis, which can be a week or two or even months? To be sure, doctors have a practical interest in not sharing every ghastly possibility before the cards are anywhere near the table. But how much pretending should go on before the diagnosis is in? How well does fiction serve the patient?

Might this be a question for the one thousand doctors at that conference to vote on? And shouldn't this be a topic of discussion—perhaps more than one!—for medical students in their version of Atul Gawande's Patient-Doctor weekly seminars?

Can I get a show of hands?

Thing Two: I Was Wrong

In October 2017, as a patient on 10 North, I walked my way to recovery, up and down the halls, mostly at night when it was quiet, admiring the people who worked there and admiring the art that filled so much wall space. Months later, during my seventeen-day "spritz" of radiation, walking through another set of the same hospital's hallways, I passed dozens more works of art—mostly fine prints, mostly bright, abstract, and sophisticated—that were donated by grateful patients. I was overjoyed to not see typical hospital art here either, and touched all over again to imagine so many talented patients who were so full of gratitude.

In 2019, in an article in the *New York Times* about the dazzling ceramic murals by Beatriz Milhazes in the entranceway to the newest wing of the hospital, I discovered how wrong I had been. There was a grander ambition at work. For ten years, the hospital has collected art—four hundred pieces by now—and it consults on acquisitions with a gallery called Salon 94. In the case of several big spaces, including a cement wall that one bank of rooms looked out onto, the hospital commissioned an artist to decorate the dreary expanse so that patients wouldn't have to stare out the window at cement.

When I walked the halls on 10 North, there had been nothing random or predictable about the artwork I saw. It was the hospital's decision to add art to the process of recovery. The hospital's decision to make a grander gesture than hanging pretty wallpaper or framing a poster or a reproduction from the Metropolitan Museum, which would have been easy enough, cheap enough—and pleasant enough. But the profusion of "real art" by contemporary artists took me by surprise. My thoughts wandered to art made in unlikely, inhospitable places—in prisons and by prisoners at Theresienstadt, the walled ghetto and Nazi concentration camp outside Prague. But I had spent no time thinking about how important it might be for a patient in a hospital to look at art until I stared at it night after solitary night, lured from my grim medical mess into someone else's vision. The pieces were easy to look at, but in no way insipid or sentimental.

The work stopped time, enough time to remind me there was something besides the IV in my arm, the uncertainty of the outcome, the gene that spooked the doctor, the actual poison dripping into my bloodstream around the clock—the poison that might lead to other cancers years from now, the sickness and sorrow behind every door I passed—and my own fear and trembling. There on the wall were shapes, colors, contrasts, and intentions that made me pause. And as touched as I had been by the idea that grateful patients had donated their artwork, I was more moved to learn that the work had been put there with such intention.

Thing Three: Sue Briskman Redux

The hospital with the art collection where Nora Ephron died and where I did not die is three blocks east of what was the Lenox School. Which returns me to the story of Sue Briskman, who died of lymphoma in 1972. Lenox was only a sliver of my life—eleventh and twelfth grades—but Sue's sickness and death took up nearly a quarter of that slender space. The two are nearly synonymous in my memory, the school and the girl who died.

After our fortieth reunion in 2012, I came to know one woman who attended the gathering. At Lenox, she and I had rarely spoken, but we've become friends, meeting for dinner once or twice a year, and we have plenty to talk about these days. She invited another classmate to our last dinner, and we met at an Indian restaurant in the East 50s. Once we'd exhausted the perfervid political discussion, when the drama was still which Democratic nominee would go up against Trump, I changed the subject: "Do you mind if I ask you about Sue Briskman? Were you traumatized by her death?"

I had asked this at the reunion a few years before, but I wondered if the answers might be different in a more intimate setting. Both women were devastated at the time—they'd known her since first grade—but, long-term, "No," said one of them without hesitation.

The other was not as sanguine. "My father died when I was in my twenties," she said, "so I'm not sure what caused what, but I worry a lot about sudden death. I walk down the street imagining the ways I could be hurt. I freak out when I have swollen lymph nodes. And I feel slightly anxious when I don't know where everyone in my family is. I don't feel entirely calm unless I'm with all of them."

Who's to say whether we're born with our jittery nervous systems or whether we acquire them once life has its way with us for a few decades? Based on the sample pool at dinner, Sue's untimely death was not an equal opportunity destabilizer. But the conversation did not end there. Though neither of these women had been her closest friend, they knew things. When she was sick, she had a boyfriend and wanted to have sex with him, and her friends either did or didn't find a way to engineer that encounter.

At the restaurant, I tried to imagine the moments around such an engagement but drew a blank. I had no idea where Sue had lived or what her state of mind—or health—could have been. Did she have any idea how sick she was? How do you tell your seventeen-year-old daughter that she's going to die soon? I vaguely remembered hearing that she grew suspicious when her parents bought her something grand for her birthday, but when had I heard that? It must have been after she died, when people were talking about how much she knew. That's my only recollection. She found the lump on her neck in 1971 and died in early 1972, four years before Susan Sontag was diagnosed with the breast cancer that would lead her to write *Illness as Metaphor*. Half a century ago. The dark ages of cancer treatment. Was it ghoulish even to imagine the scene of Sue Briskman's possible assignation? And if it happened, what about the poor boy who had been her first lover, and her last, and who had to have known that she died soon after? What must that have done to his young psyche?

"And after she died," one of my dinner companions said, "her parents got divorced."

I did not wince when I heard this, but I wince now and every time I think of it, even though I know there's a good chance neither parent is still alive. I know it's a common phenomenon after a child dies, and who knows what the state of their marriage was before Sue's sickness and death. So much can go wrong once a volcano erupts. Guilt, blame, depression, the unequal apportionment of grief between mother and father, and the dilemma of what to do with that grief. When I was young, I imagined that people in mourning would be a comfort to one another, that the comfort would be lasting and profound because the person who died had meant so much to all of them. It still seems as though that's what ought to be true, despite so much evidence to the contrary.

Thing Four: Remains

I forget about it for months and find it when I'm looking for something else—the tiny envelope of Deena's remains in my purse. *There you are. I'd nearly forgotten you were so close.* Then I say to myself: *Next time I'm by the ocean . . .* Then I say to myself: *Or maybe not. Maybe I'll just keep you right here.* Maybe, like Deena's granddaughter, I am comforted by the thought that she is always with me.

Two Years on the Nose

At the two-year-mark, in mid-December 2019, I walked into Dr. D.'s office on East 70th Street feeling wobbly about the state of my health only because I hadn't had a PET scan in eighteen months. I didn't think I had lymphoma, but I worried about the "ground glass" in my lungs: lung cancer is often asymptomatic until it's too late to treat.

The waiting room was packed as always, and once I offered my arm for a blood draw, I found an empty seat and a copy of *People*, and waited for Dr. D., with his long legs and big smile, to fetch me. Like his partner, he is a champion kibitzer and a mensch, and I sometimes have had to say to him, when we're deep into stories about summer vacations and grandchildren's college essays, "Let's talk about my health for a few minutes, OK?"

On cue, he barreled into the waiting room and greeted me warmly, like we were about to go for coffee. How am I? Have I taken any trips lately? How are the college essay kids coming along? The talk continued in the exam room, as though we *were* having coffee, my story leading to one of his and his story reminding me of the time when this happened and that happened . . . and I wondered if he developed this laissez-faire approach to put nervous patients at their ease or because he's just curious and likes to kibitz.

He finally scanned a piece of paper clipped to the front of my thick manila file and said, "The initial bloodwork is fine. I'll have the rest of the results in two or three days. Give me a call."

"And I need a PET scan, right?"

"Right. How've you been feeling?"

"Fine. Completely fine."

"Have you lost any weight?"

"No. It's very steady."

"You look fine."

He proceeded with the physical and more schmoozing about travel plans for January and his adult son and daughter, and I decided that I would wait until mid-January when I returned from a trip to Miami to get the PET scan because I didn't want to deal with the anxiety the scan kicks up during the holidays. And I wanted to enjoy Miami, especially if the scan reveals that I have, say, lung cancer.

"I'll let you know when I'm ready to schedule the PET scan," I told him as I left, because he needed to order it, but neither of us said anything about what I thought was the famous two-year mark. I knew why I hadn't—because there could be no definitive answer until the scan. But I wondered why he hadn't. Was he too waiting for the scan— or had I gotten this two-year thing wrong? Had he really said it? Had he meant it? What did it say about me that I was afraid to ask a simple question of the nicest doctor in the world?

It said that I was still a frightened ninny. One lion might have been slinking away behind me, but another one was coming right at me. Chemo and cancer had knocked my fear of flying out of me, but I was still so afraid of hearing bad news—*The two-year mark? No, it's five years before you can rest easy*—that I couldn't even ask a timing question. I was failing every lesson Deena had tried to teach me.

Two days later, when I emailed Dr. D. for the results of the additional bloodwork, I gathered the courage to clarify the timing. "I think you told me that two years with no recurrence is significant. Or did I hear that wrong? Also, you said there's now an abrogation for my terrible gene. What is it?"

Two hours later an email arrived. Bloodwork: normal. And these two brief paragraphs:

> For your type of lymphoma, the 2-year mark is significant. The majority of recurrences do occur within the first 2 years after treatment is concluded.
>
> The infusional, hospital-based treatment was given to override the adverse genetic finding. Furthermore, you had limited volume of disease. Overall, I think your prognosis is excellent.

Cue the fireworks, the marching band, the helium balloons, and a bottle of champagne. I'm dizzy with disbelief, buzzing with glee. The top of my head feels like I've already drunk the champagne—until I wonder if he's forgotten about the ground glass in my lung. Does he remember that I haven't had the PET scan? And this, my worst fear: that he's such a kibitzer, he's not paying close enough attention to every wrinkle of my medical record. Still, I run into the other room to tell James the amazing news, and I fire off happy texts to the few people I had told about the two-year mark. I'm floating a few inches off the ground. But I won't allow myself to indulge in maximum joy until I see the results of the scan. Without question, I would give Dr. D. five stars on RateMDs.com, but I have learned to measure and question and doubt what doctors tell me. I've learned that opinions, especially when swaddled in hope, count for nothing. The biopsy and the scan are king, and the rest is noise, the noise of hope and the noise of fear.

The Thing Itself and After

My first comment to the nurse checking me in for the PET scan was: "Please be sure to phone Dr. D. with the results. This is his cell number." He had given me these instructions and said he would call me with the results as soon as he heard. It was now February 25, the first appointment I could get for a scan.

"We should have the results in a day or two," she said.

I sat in a private room and drank a few quarts of a sugary mix that would help the radioactive isotopes they'd injected travel to any "avid" clusters of cells, which would "light up" on the scan. The light no one ever wants to see.

February 26, 27, and 28 came and went without a call from Dr. D. The weekend passed in silence. So did Monday, March 2. When I woke up on March 3, there was a LAB RESULT message from Weill Cornell in my email, and I sat on the edge of my couch in pajamas wondering whether to open it. I was fairly certain it would not include a note from Dr. D. explaining the report. He didn't communicate in the patient portal, and I knew the result had been sent to me automatically. I was terrified, but it was difficult not to push in a door left open a crack. I'm certain I held my breath as I clicked on "PET-CT Skull Base to Thigh-FDG."

> FINDINGS:
>> Mean liver SUV: 2.18
>> Maximum liver SUV: 2.87
>> No gross abnormalities in the visualized brain. Paranasal
> sinuses and mastoid air cells clear.
>> Normal uptake in the visualized portions of the brain,

pharyngeal lymphoid tissue, salivary glands and laryngeal musculature.

No enlarged or FDG avid lymph nodes.

Mild FDG uptake within the right thyroid gland with SUV 3.1, without corresponding nodule on CT, likely reactive.

Unchanged 1.3 cm ground-glass nodule within the right upper lobe (series 5, image 76) (SUV 1.0). Unchanged tree-in-bud nodularity within the anterior right upper lobe without hypermetabolism. No FDG avid nodules. No pleural effusion.

No enlarged or FDG avid lymph nodes.

Heart normal in size. No pericardial effusion.

The lymph node and lung situation looked good. No, they looked great! But what was the topmost finding about my liver? What did these numbers mean? Everything I Googled led to a malignancy. In. My. Liver. *Holy crap.* For instance:

Typically, a standardized uptake value (SUV), a quantity that incorporates the patient's size and the injected dose, that is more than 2.0 is considered to be suggestive of malignancy, whereas lesions with SUVs less than this value are considered to be benign.

But liver cancer? How could this be? I had no idea where my liver was, though I knew this was very bad indeed. Yet nothing hurt or felt lumpy when I pressed my abdomen. *Liver cancer.* I had licked lymphoma, clobbered incipient lung cancer—and *now I had liver cancer?* And I found out on my laptop? Was it too early to call Dr. D.? And if he'd seen this—no wonder he hadn't called me. He had to prepare to make this call. *I've got some tough news. Liver cancer.*

Jesus Christ.

James was still sleeping, but what good would it do if he were awake? The chillest man on the planet—who happened to be my husband—would not chill to this development. I reached for my phone and scrolled for Dr. D.'s cell number. It was 8:30 a.m., and I got his voicemail.

If you catch it early, is there any hope for a liver cancer patient? Any hope at all?

I Googled those two awful words and was about to click on a link when the phone rang. Dr. D.'s name flashed on the screen.

"Liz," he said, "I'm sorry I didn't call you with the results. I was out of town with a family emergency."

"I got the report in my email. It says I have liver cancer."

"*What?* No! The scan is fine."

"At the top, it says: 'Mean liver: SUV'—"

"No, no, no, that's a standard measurement. The scan is *fine.*"

"Are you sure, because—"

"The scan is perfect. You're going to live a long time! G'bye."

Goodbye!

Goodbye!

Goodbye!

And they all lived happily ever after.

The end.

I've Got a Brand-new Pair of Roller Skates

I did not have liver cancer. Or any other cancer. An hour later, I floated down Broadway to a dentist appointment, and later in the day, I went to the gym and ran around the big exercise room in the hour before the exercise classes began at 5:30 p.m., and I had to keep reminding myself that I really *really* did not have cancer of any kind, especially not lung cancer. I ran in happy circles and listened on my iPod Shuffle to Melanie singing that she had a brand new pair of roller skates, and to classic Motown and Alanis Morissette and Madonna and Cassandra Wilson and Emily playing a Beethoven string quartet, telling myself that I had to find a new way to breathe after two-and-a-half years of worry about the possibility of dying from this multiplication of cells that had taken root in me and that might take root again someday but they were not doing that now, a new way to *be*, just *be* in the world again, a new approach after a lifetime of hypochondria, of anxiety about every tiny ache, every minor upset. I would not call my sister or Zanti whenever I felt a weird flutter, a random twinge. I was so beyond that, having been all the way to the chemo ward and back, to Vietnam and back.

Now could I say I was mellow? Was I chill? Or just relieved and happy? And this happiness could power a kite. A car. A weekend in the sun. When I got home, I would check the hotel in Miami where we like to stay and find out the room rates if I went in a few days, for a few days. Just to relax by the water. Walk for miles on the beach. A celebration. A splurge. A few days when I could be as buoyant as a bouquet of helium balloons. *I was going to live a long time!*

At home on the computer screen in my lap, the hotel rooms in Miami were $279—a bit steep for my budget—and on the TV screen across the room was the news, a mashup of numbers and warnings that I had been monitoring in the previous days and weeks but could focus on now with more clarity because I had one less worry than I'd had the night before. The numbers were climbing, and the voices of the broadcasters approaching panic. I had been paying attention— because that's what hypochondriacs *do*—to news from Wuhan, from Italy, and from the coast of California, where a cruise ship full of infected people had been forced to linger in the water beyond the San Francisco Bay, and I knew the virus was coming our way, but we had some time. On February 25, I'd ordered a hundred surgical masks— for an already jacked-up price of $130—that would be delivered any day. Emily was expected in our apartment the next afternoon for a few days of rehearsals, and I would give her a stack of masks and a bag of the latex gloves I'd bought in a hardware store.

I was sure it would inch across the country, West to East, state by state, and arrive in New York in three or four weeks, and by then, we'd have our supplies, and in the meantime, every time I went out, I bought chicken to freeze and a few cans of tuna. And I kept my eye on the hotel rates in Miami. If they took a big dip, I might hop on a plane one of these days.

Breaking News

BREAKING NEWS: W.H.O. CONFIRMS
90K COVID CASES WORLDWIDE

BREAKING NEWS: CDC: "US PAST
CONTAINMENT POINT"

BREAKING NEWS: Emily's rehearsal is canceled because her up-coming concert is canceled. She is bypassing New York City on her way home from a concert tour in Florida. I cannot give her the gloves or the masks or the list of Virus Warning Signs. I don't want to frighten her, but I want her to know what to do, just in case. I read that zinc lozenges might be good for fighting this, so I ordered a supply, but I'll have to mail them to her when they come.

Voices of newscasters grow more insistent as they report climbing numbers and growing fears. Miami hotel rates sink, but so does my plan to go there or anywhere else, including outside. One afternoon, Nancy calls with stark news. Her husband, who works at Columbia University, just finished a conference call with news from the governor: in the next twenty-four to forty-eight hours, he'll issue a stay-at-home order, and my sweet dreams of the virus hopscotching leisurely across the country and arriving weeks from now were as wrong as the doctors who kept telling me I didn't have cancer. In fact, the damn virus took the red-eye from San Francisco to New York and missed flyover country completely.

Within minutes of Nancy's phone call, James and I head out with separate shopping lists, he to the drugstore and I to Fairway and

Zabar's for as much as we can carry without looking like we're about to board the last plane out of Lisbon in 1941. On my way home, I stop at a small pharmacy where I once noticed a shelf of CBD gummies. I'd never had the slightest interest in trying them, but that afternoon, I buy a bottle because I am more anxious than I have been since . . . since the moment I found the lump in my armpit. Since the moment the doctor told me I was positive for a gene that meant I might not respond to treatment. This new threat is my own terror, inflated to the size of a mushroom cloud.

Is everyone schlepping up and down Broadway with grocery bags as anxious—as frightened to death—as I am? Some of us are wearing masks, so expressions are hard to read, but those already making that fashion statement, even if their sisters haven't called with dire plans from the governor's office, must be paying as much attention as I am to the news. But a friend intends to board a plane in the morning for Europe, to play chamber music in beautiful halls where the sounds of his instrument will fill rooms with joy, transcendence, maybe even hope. By the end of the day, his concerts are canceled, and dominoes are falling in every direction. I call a friend who is getting a degree in education and teaches part-time in New York City schools, to find out if she's still working. She tells me the mayor has decided to close the schools but doesn't know when he'll announce it.

"How do you know?" I ask.

"A friend heard it from a Department of Education official in the steam room at the Harvard Club."

When I laugh out loud, she laughs too, and we're both so keyed up that our laughter explodes because we know this might be the funniest thing we'll hear for a long time. Otherwise, we tiptoe around, making small gestures, wondering what to do next, hungry for news and terrified of it at the same time. In almost every conversation, clichés abound. *The world as we know it, the world turned upside down, we've entered the twilight zone.*

How Are You Holding Up?

On the plus side, it was not long before I realized that a lifetime of hypochondria had prepared me for this, along with two and a half years of cancer fear, cancer tests, cancer denial, cancer itself, cancer treatment, and now—drumroll!—cancer survival. As when I was sick, the casual question, "How are you?" seemed wildly inappropriate. And the routine answer, "Fine, how are you?" was now a laugh line. Instead, I said to friends, "How are you holding up?" which implied a base level of difficulty—shared fear, disbelief, and anger. And I expected to hear more grim candor in their answers than the question usually generated, even from the most optimistic.

Something else familiar from my illness: the way time stood still in the early quarantine weeks, or whatever it did that took so long to adjust to. The door slamming on the events, encounters, and activities that organize a life, and all of those gaps wrapped in fear. The worm at the core had come for all of us.

New York was the epicenter, and we weren't sure it was safe to take the elevator and breathe at the same time. I could hold my breath from the first floor to the fifth but not the ninth, where I live. Those early weeks reminded me of all the mornings I woke up when I was afraid I had cancer and when I knew I had it and felt I had nothing to look forward to but counting the hours until I could go to sleep again because *my life as I knew it was over, and it might never come back.* That the dread was familiar didn't make going through it again any easier, except I could entertain the possibility that *my life as I knew it* might one day return, because it once had. Still, I had to remind myself that, according to the scariest, most reliable, and penetrating scan—taken by a machine that sees into my cells—I was fine. In no uncertain terms. No opinions. No euphemisms. No cheery hopes from doctors who don't like to give us bad news. I. Was. Fine.

The rest of the world was not.

Good News, Bad News

With my bright, shiny bill of health, I could finally figure out how to write my memoir, this memoir. I had a clearer idea of what sort of cancer memoir it would be, of what my relationship would be to the material, to the story. It was news I had waited on for years, news that made me rejoice—except that the dark cloud of Covid-19 had just engulfed all of us. Almost overnight, my assignment had changed: write about surviving cancer in the midst of a global pandemic. It was like having to learn two new languages at the same time—Russian and Chinese. When I mentioned the dilemma to a writer friend, she said calmly, "Put your manuscript in a drawer until this is over." That was when we thought it might last a few weeks, a month on the outside.

I did what she said for four months and then returned to these pages. I rewrote, rearranged, and reimagined. It took much longer to find the right words in the right order than I hoped it would. But it always does. When I wasn't working on it, I wrote essays for *Salma-*

gundi and kept a Covid diary that was published in the magazine in late 2020. It was hard to find my way back to writing fiction when real life was so full of apocalyptic narratives—not just one but several. But that, as they say, is another story.

Dress Rehearsal

I had the luxury of something other than a terminal diagnosis, the luxury of only one bad gene that might nix my treatment and that, three years later, does not appear to have nixed it after all. For all the comments doctors made, not one of them said, "It's time to get your affairs in order," but at different times over many months, the worm and I were eye to eye. Our proximity made me nauseated, made me curl up on the couch and cry, wake up in the middle of the night seized with terror, and want to scream when people asked me how I was. The only thing I did not do was sleep with the lights on.

I knew someone who went to the farewell party that F. Scott and Zelda Fitzgerald's daughter Frances had for herself in 1986 when she knew she was dying. I did not have to contemplate planning such a party for myself. Not yet.

I have a friend whose mother gathered her eight grown children together to say goodbye before she downed a bottle of barbiturates prescribed for the purpose by her doctor in a state where that's permitted.

When James' sister was going into her fifth year of stage four lung cancer, getting a regular dose of chemo at Dana Farber, she ran into a nurse she knew. "You!" the nurse exclaimed. "You were supposed to die years ago!" Probably not in the nurse's Handbook of Thoughtful

Phrases, but death and dying do that. It's not only patients who suffer from brain fog.

I wonder—perhaps as often as others do—if James and I will have the luxury to decide when and how we will die or the courage to take matters into our own hands if we have the choice. I hope we will be lucky and brave and not be terrible burdens on our loved ones.

I hope what everyone else hopes: not today, not now, not anytime soon.

This time, I did not have to get my affairs in order, did not have to make out a list of my passwords (God help me), or face the ultimate fear of not being, but one day I will have to. If I'm *compos mentis*, it will require mettle and nerves I did not have to exercise in the last few years.

Can it be that this illness was a dress rehearsal for whatever crisis comes next, and that next time I will be less like myself and more like Deena? Ask more questions and be less afraid of the answers? Will I remember the lessons that Dr. Gawande learned and resist the cowering that came so naturally to me?

If at all possible, I will let you know.

Plot Twists

Cancer-wise, I'm still fine and, twenty-four months into Covid-19, fine too, as are the people I love most, but the planet is wrapped in an enormous blanket of isolation, fear, and ever-changing mask, medical, and vaccine advice, deadly variants, less deadly variants, and political polarization at home and abroad. Yet as grave as the situation is,

I can't help but note, with a speck of amusement, that I am no longer alone in my hypochondria. Caution and vulnerability are the new normal. This story does not exactly end with me getting all the way over my hyper-anxiety, but with the world itself providing an unexpected plot twist: seven billion people are keeping me company with *their* anxiety and travel constraints. Virus and vaccine news punctuates—when it doesn't dominate—newscasts and conversations.

In another plot twist, my one-woman fear-of-flying club has many new members. They're not afraid of planes falling out of the sky, as I was, but of unruly passengers and conflicts over vaccine mandates and mask-wearing at 35,000 feet. Flight attendants are slugged and end up hospitalized. A passenger who couldn't control himself was duct-taped to a seat. A first-class passenger decked a flight attendant because, allegedly, she brushed against him as she walked by. She apologized but, according to news reports, he decked her anyway. So it goes.

And in a final plot twist as I work my way to the end of this story, I woke up on a recent morning and decided to do something I have wanted to do for a very long time, but with so many Covid restrictions, I was not sure how to manage. I called the doctor who took care of me once I was diagnosed, the man who suggested I write a book about people with red hair. The man whose baritone voice told me three-and-a-half-years ago that I was cured except for the gene that spooked him.

"The doctor is with a patient," the receptionist said. "What is it you want to talk to him about?"

"I was his patient, and I'm writing a book, and I need to ask him some questions."

"Your name?"

After I said my name, I said, "And please write this next to my name," and I told her the name of the gene. "He'll know who I am." The last time I had seen him was passing by in his office several years before, no longer his patient. I had said hello and, looking at me, he said the name of the gene and, "The problem was under your right arm."

The phone rang ten minutes later, and I explained why I was calling. "I was too afraid to ask you anything when I was your patient, but I'm writing a book, and I need to know what you would have told me if I had been brave enough to ask you why you were so spooked by my gene."

"What I would have told you is that if you have an abnormality in that gene, the prognosis generally isn't as good as those who have a normal gene. However, that doesn't mean you can't have a good response, but fewer people do as well. The fact that you've gone three years without a recurrence is great. And if you've gone three years without any treatment and you're free of disease, that bespeaks a very good prognosis because most relapses occur within three years, and relapses after three years are mostly in the single digits. Chances of relapse are less than ten percent."

"If I had a recurrence, what would you do?"

"We would use some of the new techniques that have come out. CAR-T and bispecific antibodies. We have a whole bunch of new things. Things that would override the abnormal gene."

"New since 2017?"

"Yes."

"It's not like I would die immediately?"

"No, we have a lot of things, but it's more complicated if you relapse after having been in remission. But the longer you go, the better the prognosis. Even if you were to relapse later, those people who relapse later do better than those who relapse quickly. Take some comfort. You may very well be cured."

"Was I born with this abnormality?"

"No, I'm sure it's acquired."

"Is that why I got lymphoma?"

"No, it characterizes your lymphoma, but it doesn't tell us why you got it. . . . Yes, I remember you very well. The lymph node was under your right arm. Don't ask me what I had for breakfast, but that I remember. I remember what floor you were on. You were on the tenth floor, in that three-bedded room on 10 North."

There were only two beds in that room when I was there, and it's hard to imagine where a third would fit, but he must have remembered a period when there were three. My great good fortune is that he—and his thousand colleagues—haven't been wrong yet.

Another Plot Twist

As I reach the finish line, I pause one morning to scan the *New York Times*, and nearly knock over my coffee when I find the headline, "Women are Calling Out 'Medical Gaslighting'" (March 28, 2022) and the subhead: "Studies show female patients and people of color are more likely to have their symptoms dismissed by medical providers. Experts say: Keep asking questions."

Deena lives.

It Doesn't Come Down to Lessons, But . . .

The trick is to find the right balance between feeling too much fear and not enough to protect yourself from danger.

Silence is not merely the absence of sound. It might be rage, fear, exhaustion, prayer, or grief. It might be all of them or just a few. It might be the wordless response to catastrophe or the wordless response to beauty. At the end of certain plays or pieces of music, the audience leaps to their feet with applause. At the end of others, rarely, they are too moved to clap.

Adaptation is a biological process by which organisms or species become better suited to their environments. By which I mean that going gray, Zoom, facemasks, and *Living with Cancer* are now features of everyday life, when they would have been unimaginable a mere three years ago.

Many studies on happiness find that individuals who exercise daily, do things for others, and take regular note of what they have to be grateful for are happier than those who don't.

Years after her cancer diagnosis in 1975, Susan Sontag wrote, "I am gleaming with survivorship."

For today, for now, I know what she means.

Acknowledgments

This final note is another sort of memoir. It's a pleasure to recall the many people who had a hand in this project and a great sorrow to think of those no longer here to be thanked: Deena Kolbert, Michael Downing, Judith Hillman Paterson, and Daniel Dolgin.

In 2022, Suleika Jaouad asked me to write about hair for her *Isolation Journals*, some years after I asked her to write about hair for *Me, My Hair and I*. Carmen Radley's inspired editing of that piece about chemo hair was an important influence in a late draft of this book.

Many friends and colleagues helped along the way. Kate Hough and John Hough were insistent that I write this book when I was not sure I could or should. They were patient readers of early drafts as were Mark Bomster, Robert Boyers, Cynthia Jabs, Gail Kinn, Sue Lehmann, Stephen McCauley, Amit Pandya, Evelyn Toynton, and Charlie Peters. Michael Wood reminded me that this would take time, and he was right. Gabrielle Glaser got me through some rough patches. As always, Jesse Kornbluth's advice was spot on. Karen Karbo breathed friendship and life into me and this project when I needed both. Stephan Kolbert and Ingrid Marcroft offered information and insights into Deena that I cherish along with their friendship.

The friends and family who called, listened, brought food, sent flowers, and sustained and cheered me up mean more than I will ever be able to say.

In another category entirely are the excellent doctors I was fortunate to find, among them Dr. Morton Coleman, Dr. Julian Decter, and Dr. Evan Leibu. Much gratitude always to Dr. Charles Kellner. I hope Joyce Hackett won't mind one last, large, public thank you.

And in yet another category, I'm grateful to the amazing students I work with every day, who inspire me with their smarts, ambitions, and ability to do multivariable calculus.

It's hard to imagine publishers as conscientious and kind as Robert Mandel, Dena Mandel, and Merrill Leffler; a copy editor as diligent as Mary Beth Hinton; and the artful eyes and talents of Sophie Appel and Barbara Werden. I have a lifetime of gratitude to bestow on Gail Hochman, Marianne Merola, and the team at Brandt & Hochman.

And this is the place to say thank you from the bottom and the top of my heart to Zanti, Evelyn, Nancy, Emily, Julia, and James.